Mapping of the Brain

Faisal R. Jahangiri

MD, CNIM, DABNM, FASNM, FASET

Copyright © 2021 Global Innervation LLC

All rights reserved.

ISBN: 9798700754903

DEDICATION

To my parents, wife, children, siblings and teachers.

CONTENTS

Acknowledgments   i

1   **Mapping of the Sensory Cortex**   1

2   **Mapping of the Motor Cortex**   17

3   **Mapping of the Language Cortex**   41

ACKNOWLEDGMENTS

I want to acknowledge all my students at the Department of Neuroscience, School of Behavioral and Brain Science, The University of Texas at Dallas, Richardson, Texas. Everyone worked very hard to make this book possible.

CHAPTER 1

MAPPING OF THE SENSORY CORTEX

Faisal R. Jahangiri[1,2,3], Katharine Pautler[1],

Keri Watters[1], Sahar S. Anjum[1], Gabrielle L. Bennett[1]

[1]The University of Texas at Dallas

[2]Global Innervation LLC

[3]Axis Neuromonitoring LLC

ABSTRACT

Intraoperative sensory cortical mapping is a reliable and safe method for the central sulcus' functional localization (CS). It is utilized during neurosurgical procedures performed near eloquent brain tissue. It helps in identifying the somatosensory cortex and CS, hence preventing any postoperative neurological deficits. When executed correctly, this method can identify the somatosensory cortex for both the upper and lower limbs by locating the CS. This technical report outlines the benefits of cortical sensory mapping (CsM) and detailed methodology. With the help of a properly trained intraoperative neuromonitoring staff who can accurately interpret the signals being monitored, CsM can help in injury prevention during brain surgeries.

Keywords: cortical sensory mapping, sensory cortex, ssep, somatosensory evoked potentials, ionm, neurophysiology, intraoperative neuromonitoring

INTRODUCTION

The surgical procedures involving the resection of lesions located near or within the central sulcus (CS) increase the risk of postoperative neurological deficits. Motor and sensory functions in the contralateral face, upper, and lower extremities are a few of the major concerns. A multimodality intraoperative neurophysiological monitoring (IONM) with cortical sensory mapping (CsM) and cortical motor mapping (CmM) is a well-published method for the identification of the CS. The accurate identification of the CS and the eloquent tissue in the exposed cortex can decrease the risk of any postoperative neurological deficits [1]. The IONM provides more accurate functional and real-time intraoperative feedback to the surgeon than preoperative magnetoencephalography (MEG) and functional magnetic resonance imaging (fMRI). The CsM is vital in assuring quality outcomes of surgeries affecting the eloquent tissue of the brain. This mapping technique is utilized to identify the CS, postcentral, and pre-central gyri and record from the sensory cortex to ensure that the sensory pathway has not been affected by surgical practices [2].

Monitoring sensory functioning while performing a procedure on the somatosensory cortex is essential to minimize sensory function loss, prevent accidental clipping of a critical vessel, and prevent lesions to important brain regions [3]. The CsM can be utilized during the surgical procedure involving but not limited to epilepsy, arteriovenous malformations (AVM), aneurysms, embolism, and brain tumors. AVM only leads to symptomology in approximately 12%, with neurological AVMs typically resulting in more adverse effects. A small portion, only 4%, of AVMs result in hemorrhage, and the risk of "steal" effect or lack of oxygen to the brain also exists. Sometimes to treat this, a surgeon may implement sclerotherapy and embolization. Both these procedures may possess a risk of neural damage. Thus, cortical mapping can reduce these risks by accurately identifying the CS, sensory, and motor cortex [4]. In surgical resection of the brain tumor, the CsM may be used to locate pre-central and postcentral gyri both preoperatively and intraoperatively. This methodology allows for localization of the sensorimotor cortex via somatosensory evoked potentials (SSEP) monitoring showing a success rate of 92%. However, limitations exist in tumor resection of peri-rolandic masses [5].

TECHNICAL REPORT

Anesthesia

Total intravenous anesthesia (TIVA) is a preferred recommended anesthesia technique for CsM. If the patient is intubated, a train of four (TOF) monitoring should be performed from the most distal muscle.

Intraoperative neurophysiological monitoring

After intubation, the patient is placed in a supine position with the head turned either right (left side tumor) or left (right side tumor) and fixed with the operating table with pins in a Mayfield frame. Surface adhesive electrodes are placed for stimulation of upper and lower limb SSEPs. For upper limb SSEP stimulation, the electrodes were placed at the wrist for ulnar nerve (UN) and median nerve (MN) and at the medial ankle for the posterior tibial nerve (PTN).

For the MN setup, the ground is placed on the palmar surface of the forearm. The stimulating cathode is placed between the tendons of the palmaris longus and flexor carpi radialis tendons, 2 cm proximal to the wrist's crease. The anode is placed 2-3 cm distal to the cathode on the palmar surface [6]. For the UN stimulation, the cathode is placed 2-4 cm proximal to the wrist crease on the side of the flexor carpi ulnaris. The anode is placed 2 3 cm distal to the cathode, and the ground is placed on the forearm's palmar surface. The ground for the PTN is placed on the calf. The cathode is placed at the ankle midway between the Achilles tendon's medial border and the posterior border of the medial malleolus. The anode is placed 2-3 cm distal to the cathode [3, 6].

The subdermal needle electrodes are placed according to the international 10-20 system guidelines for recording the upper and lower limbs SSEPs at FPz, CPz, CP3, CP4, Cv5 (fifth cervical spine), EP (left and right Erb points), and PF (popliteal fossa) [7]. The baseline SSEP should be recorded after intubation and before incision. The MN stimulation intensity: 25-30 milliamperes (mA), pulse width (PW): 300 microseconds (μs), and repetition rate (RR): 2-5 per second. The UN stimulation intensity: 15-25 mA, PW: 300 μs, and RR: 2-5 per second. The PTN stimulation intensity: 45-75 mA, PW: 300 μs, and RR: 2-5 per second. The bandpass filter includes a 30 Hz low-frequency filter (LFF) and a 3000 Hz high-frequency filter (HFF) with a sweep of 100 milliseconds and 20-50 averages.

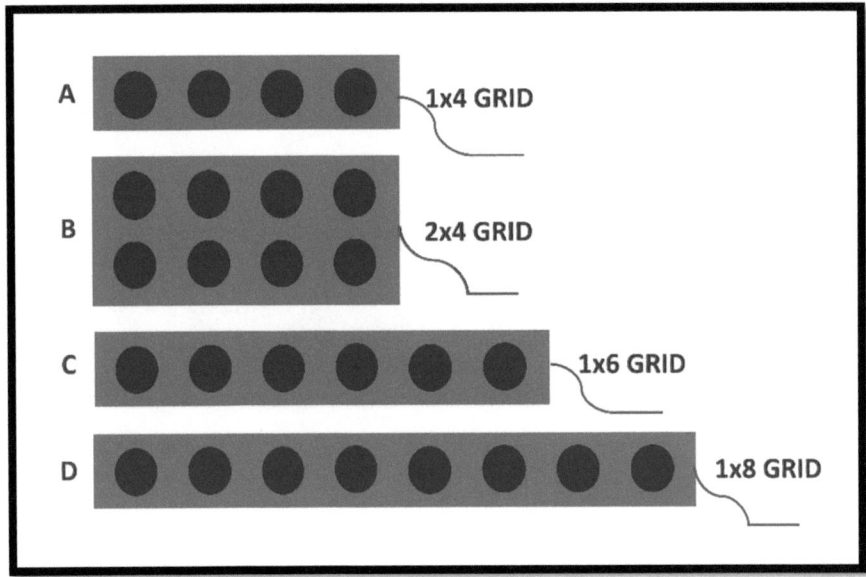

Figure 1: Cortical grids. Schematic presentation of the cortical grids. A: four-contact grid (1 x 4); B: eight contact grid (2 x 4); C: six-contact grid (1 x 6); and D: eight-contact grid (1 x 8)

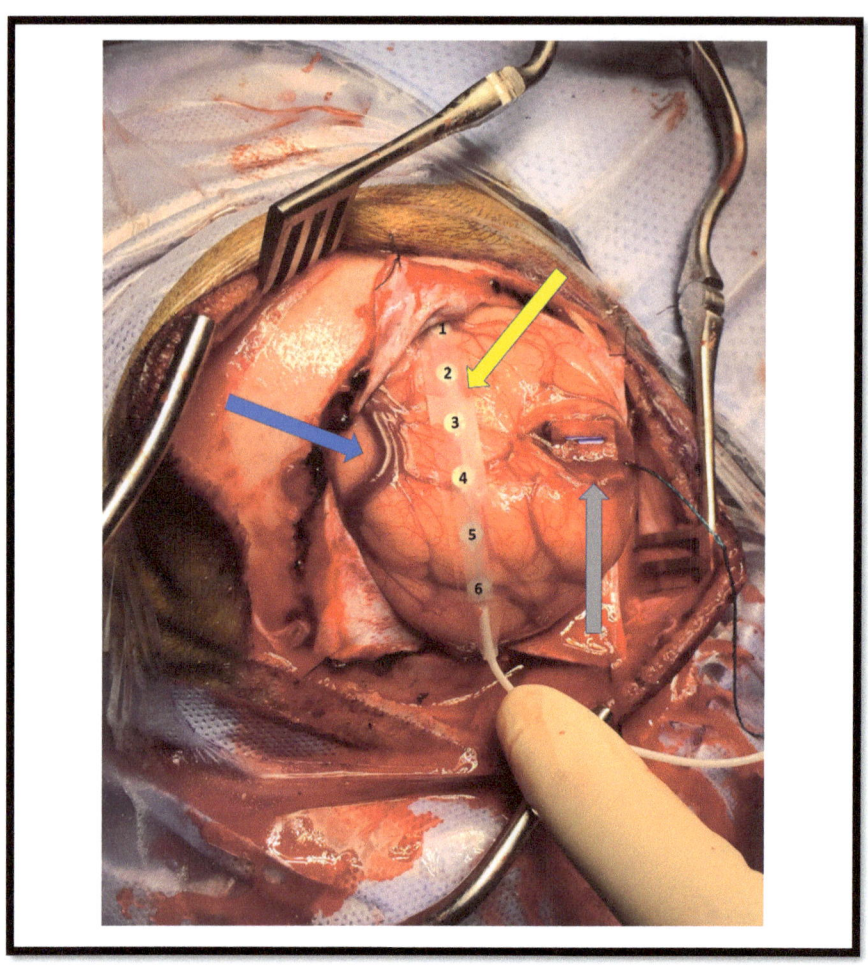

Figure 2: Grid placement for PR. A photograph of the exposed brain after opening the dura. A six contact (1 x 6) grid was placed on the cortex (yellow arrow), omega (blue arrow), and the tumor (gray arrow). PR, phase reversal

The CsM with phase reversal (PR) is performed by stimulating the contralateral ulnar, median, and PTN are recording from the ipsilateral cortical surface. After the cerebral cortex is exposed adequately, a subdural electrode grid made of stainless steel or platinum disc electrodes embedded in flexible silicone is placed on the cortical surface (Figures 1-3). A subdural grid with eight-contacts (2 x 4) (Figure 1) is placed where the CS is assumed to be for waveform interpretation [8]. Depending upon the exposed cortex's location and tumor size, an alternate size grid can be placed (1 x 4, 1 x 6, or 1 x 8). The electrodes should not be floating in a pool of blood, CSF, or irrigating solution.

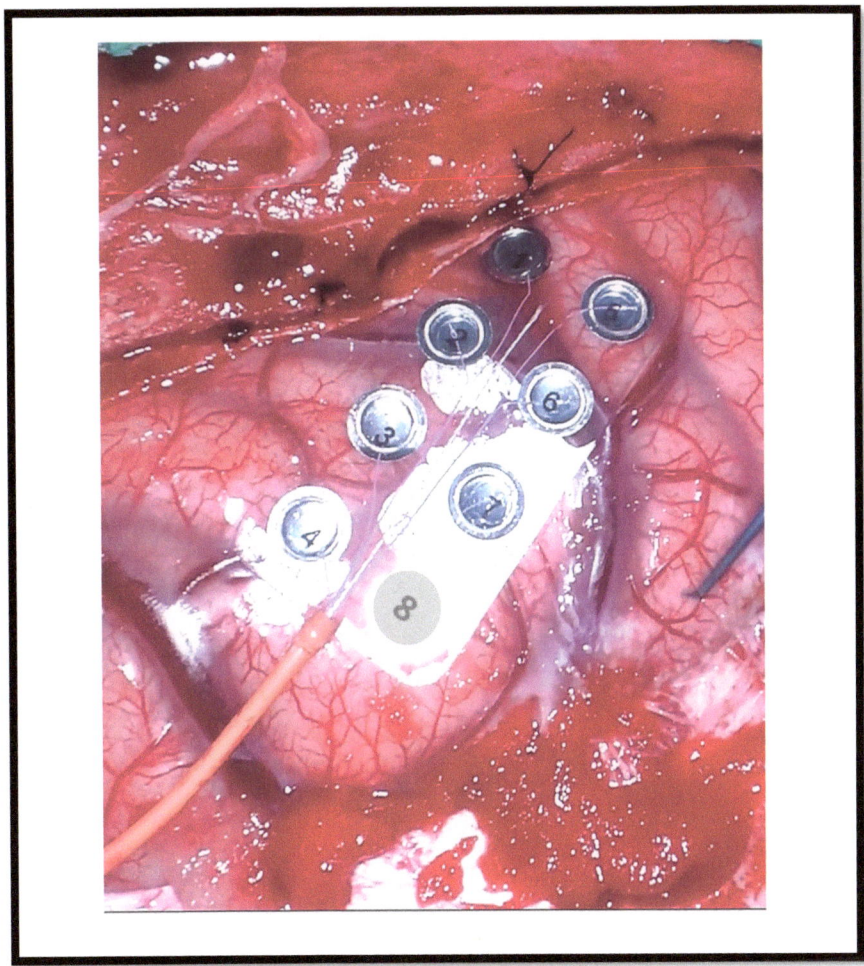

Figure 3: Grid placement for Phase Reversal (PR). An exposed part of the brain after opening the dura. An eight contact (2 x 4) grid is placed on the cerebral cortex.

The referential recordings taken from grid contacts over the precentral and postcentral gyri produce a median and UN PR between the N20 and P20 (Figure 4). This PR allows the ability to locate the CS between the two contacts. If the exposed cortex is situated posterior to the CS, all the responses will be postcentral with negative upward peaks (N20). If the exposed cortex is located anterior to the CS, all the responses will be pre-central with positive downward peaks (P20). If an apparent PR is not seen, then the contact with the largest amplitude of the N20 and P20 waveforms gives the general location of the CS. If the tumor is near the midline close to lower limb representation on the cerebral cortex, CsM with the PTN is performed. A PR is rarely recorded for PTN. The location of the CS is either directly beneath or a few millimeters anterior or posterior to the area of the largest P37/N45 wave amplitude (Figure 5).

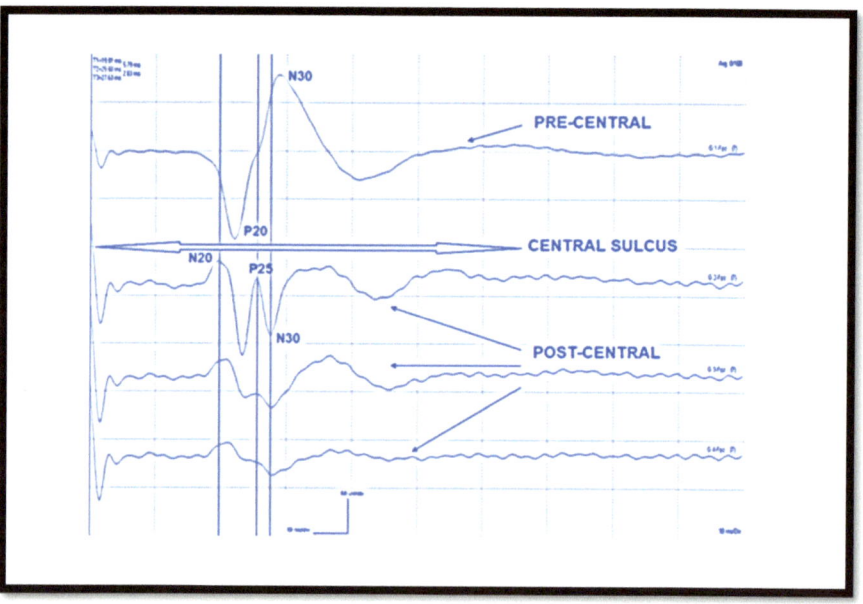

Figure 4: On-axis mapping with P25. On-axis MN sensory mapping by a 1x4 grid with a triphasic phase reversal, including a P25 response. The PR is between G1 and G2. The response from

G1 is pre-central, and G2, G3, and G4 are postcentral. MN, median nerve; PR, phase reversal.

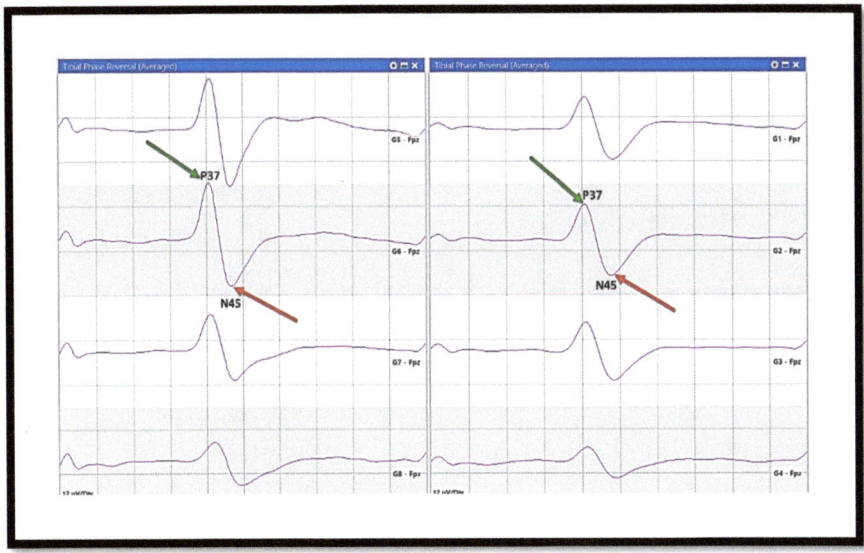

Figure 5: PTN sensory mapping. A PTN sensory mapping by a 2 x 4 grid. The PR is not present. The CS is localized by the largest amplitude responses (P37 peak) from G2 and G6. A large positive P37 peak (green arrow) and a large negative N45 peak (red arrow). PTN, posterior tibial nerve; PR, phase reversal; CS, central sulcus

DISCUSSION

Mapping for the sensorimotor cortex is typically done for tumors located in the frontal or parietal lobes, and within or encroaching upon the sensorimotor areas. The patient is usually under general anesthesia. Dependent upon the location desired for mapping, different nerves are utilized. Upper extremities require median or UNs, whereas lower extremities rely on the PTN [9].

These procedures should be mapped using both SSEPs recorded from the postcentral sensory cortex to identify the CS and direct cortical motor evoked potentials (dcMEP) stimulation to identify the motor cortex. The localization of the CS is the first step in identifying the pre-central and postcentral gyri. If the motor gyrus is outside the tumor resection area, further motor mapping may not be needed. The PR is a phenomenon due to the opposite polarity of the direct cortical SSEP (dcSSEP) signals recorded across the CS.

The CS is about halfway between the rostral and caudal poles of the hemispheres. This sulcus divides the frontal lobe in the rostral half of the hemisphere from the more caudal parietal lobe [10]. The utilization of CsM by stimulating contralateral MN, UN, and PTN may be used to identify the CS. The tumor could potentially push the CS, either anterior, posterior, medial, or lateral. Although the CS varies in how it physically looks from person to person, there are

general landmarks that can help distinguish it from other structures surrounding it. The sigmoidal hook, where the pre-central gyrus bulges posteriorly, also known as the omega sign, is a feature of the CS.

If the grid electrode is not placed accurately over the CS, it may result in an off-axis mapping represented as the traditional dual-radial model (Figure 6) [11]. This may result in the misinterpretation of the results [1]. The on-axis mapping is performed by continuing the PR until tangential-radial triphasic (TRT) peaks (N20/P25/P30) is recorded from the postcentral gyrus (Figure 7). The TRT cortical SSEP model generates two dipoles. The first tangential dipole generates the N20 and P20 peaks across the CS, and the second dipole generates a radially oriented P25 peak in the CS [8]. Depending on the surgery, the use of IONM with accurate CsM can offer greater accuracy of the identification of the CS and somatosensory cortex. This may decrease with varying degrees of postoperative neurological deficits. A false negative interpretation may occur if the grid contacts are above a large tumor and do not record any responses.

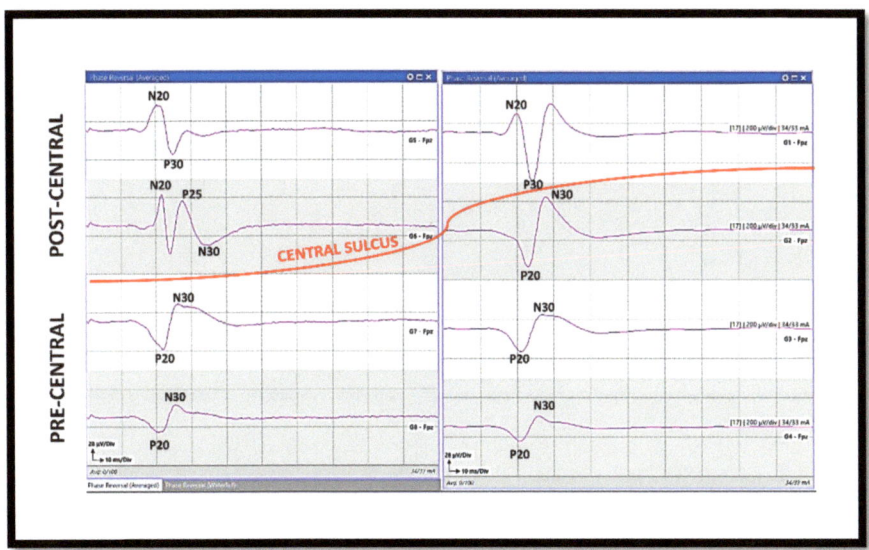

Figure 6: Off-axis mapping. Incomplete on-axis (off-axis) MN sensory mapping by a 2 x 4 grid with a triphasic PR, including a P25 response. The PR is between G1/G2 and G6/G7 localizing the CS (red line). The responses from G1, G5, and G6 are postcentral, and G2, G3, G4, G7, and G8 are pre-central. MN, median nerve; PR, phase reversal; CS, central sulcus

Other mapping techniques such as fMRI and MRI exist; however, they are not as portable as CsM. These methods also may not be as economical or practical for surgical use. Some possible pathologies that may require CsM include cerebral aneurysm, AVM, and intracranial tumors [12-13].

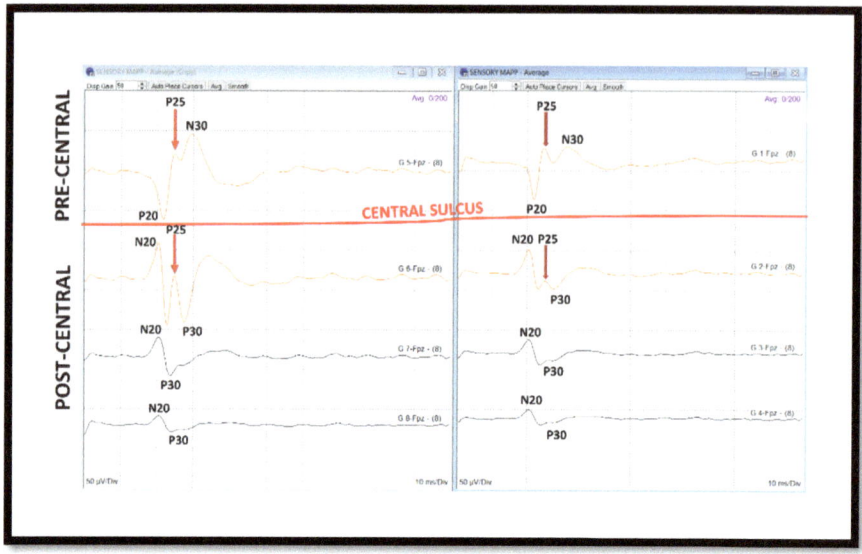

Figure 7: On-axis mapping. An on-axis MN sensory mapping by a 2 x 4 grid with a triphasic PR, including a P25 response. The PR is between G1/G2 and G5/G6 localizing the CS (red line). The responses from G1 and G5 are pre-central, and G2, G3, G4, G7, and G8 are postcentral. MN, median nerve; PR, phase reversal; CS, central sulcus.

CONCLUSIONS

Intraoperative neurophysiological sensory cortical mapping with the N20/P20 or N20/P25/P30 PR of the SSEPs is a safe, reliable, helpful technique to identify the CS. It provides a better understanding of the spatial location and functionality of the cortical region.

The neurophysiologist's experience and the operating surgeon involved is a crucial factor is successful cortical mapping. The cortical mapping helps the surgeon intraoperatively to identify the CS and differentiate the sensory and motor cortex. Multimodality cortical mapping should be performed when the motor function is at risk and may result in any postoperative neurological deficits.

DISCLOSURES

Human subjects: Consent was obtained by all participants in this study. **Animal subjects:** All authors have confirmed that this study did not involve animal subjects or tissue. **Conflicts of interest:** In compliance with the ICMJE uniform disclosure form, all authors declare the following: **Payment/services info:** All authors have declared that no financial support was received from any organization for the submitted work. **Financial relationships:** All authors have declared that they have no financial relationships at present or within the previous three years with any organizations that might have an interest in the submitted work. **Other relationships:** All authors have declared that there are no other relationships or activities that could appear to have influenced the submitted work.

REFERENCES

1. Wood CC, Spencer DD, Allison T, McCarthy G, Williamson PD, Goff WR: Localization of human sensorimotor cortex during surgery by cortical surface recording of somatosensory evoked potentials. J Neurosurg. 1988, 68:99-111.

2. Passmore SR, Murphy B, Lee TD: The origin, and application of somatosensory evoked potentials as a neurophysiological technique to investigate neuroplasticity. J Can Chiropr Assoc. 2014, 58:170-183.

3. Toleikis JR: Intraoperative monitoring using somatosensory evoked potentials. A position statement by the American Society of Neurophysiological Monitoring. J Clin Monit Comput. 2005, 19:241-258. 10.1007/s10877-005-4397-0

4. Arteriovenous Malformations. (2019). Accessed: Nov 20, 2019: https://www.hopkinsmedicine.org/health/conditions-and-diseases/arteriovenous-malformations.

5. Romstöck J, Fahlbusch R, Ganslandt O: Localisation of the sensorimotor cortex during surgery for brain tumours: feasibility and waveform patterns of somatosensory evoked potentials. J Neurol Neurosurg Psychiatry. 2002, 72:221-229. 10.1136/jnnp.72.2.221

6. Jahangiri FR: Surgical Neurophysiology. Jahangiri FR (ed): CreateSpace, North Carolina; 2012.

7. Acharya JN, Hani A, Cheek J, Thirumala P, Tsuchida TN: American Clinical Neurophysiology Society Guideline 2: Guidelines for standard electrode position nomenclature. J Clin Neurophysiol. 2016, 33:308-311. 10.1097/WNP.0000000000000316

8. Jahangiri FR, Sherman JH, Sheehan J, Shaffrey M, Dumont AS, Vengrow M, Vega-Bermudez F: Limiting the current density during localization of the primary motor cortex by using a tangential-radial cortical somatosensory evoked potentials model, direct electrical cortical stimulation, and electrocorticography. Neurosurgery. 2011, 69:893-898. 10.1227/NEU.0b013e3182230ac3

9. Stecker MM: A review of intraoperative monitoring for spinal surgery. Surg Neurol Int. 2012, 3:S174-S187. 10.4103/2152-7806.98579

10. Purves D, Augustine GJ, Fitzpatrick D, Hall WC, LaMantia A-S, McNamara JO, Williams SM: Neuroscience Third Edtion. Purves D, Augustine GJ, Fitzpatrick D, Hall WC, LaMantia A-S, McNamara JO, Williams SM (ed): Sinauer, Massachusetts; 2004.

11. Cedzich C, Taniguchi M, Schäfer S, Schramm J: Somatosensory evoked potential phase reversal and direct motor cortex stimulation during surgery in and around the central region. Neurosurgery. 1996, 38:962-970. 10.1097/00006123-199605000-00023

12. Husain AM: A Practical Approach to Neurophysiologic Intraoperative Monitoring. Husain AM (ed): Demos Medical, New York; 2014.

13. Chiong W, Leonard MK, Chang EF: Neurosurgical patients as human research subjects: Ethical considerations in intracranial electrophysiology research Neurosurgery. Neurosurgery. 2018, 83:29-37.

Citation:

Jahangiri FR, Pautler K, Watters K, Anjum SS, Bennett GL. Mapping of the Somatosensory Cortex. Cureus. 2020 Mar 19;12(3):e7332. doi: 10.7759/cureus.7332. PMID: 32313773; PMCID: PMC7164708.

CHAPTER 2

MAPPING OF THE MOTOR CORTEX

Faisal R. Jahangiri[1,2,3], Aksharkumar Dobariya[1], Aaron Kruse[1], Olga Kalyta[1], John D. Moorman[1]

The University of Texas at Dallas

Global Innervation LLC

Axis Neuromonitoring LLC

ABSTRACT

The resection of brain tumors located within or near the eloquent tissue has a higher risk of postoperative neurological deficits. The primary concerns include loss of sensory and motor functions in the contralateral face, upper and lower extremities, as well as speech deficits. Intraoperative neurophysiological monitoring (IONM) techniques are performed routinely for the identification and preservation of the functional integrity of the eloquent brain areas during neurosurgical procedures. The IONM modalities involve sensory, motor, and language mapping, which helps in the identification of the boundaries of these areas during surgical resection. Cortical motor Mapping (CmM) technique is considered as a gold-standard technique for mapping of the brain. We present the intraoperative CmM technique, including anesthesia recommendations, types of electrodes, as well as stimulation and recording parameters for successful monitoring.

Keywords: Brain tumor, neurosurgery, motor mapping, cortical mapping, IONM, EEG, neuro-monitoring, electrocorticography.

INTRODUCTION

The first documented cortical tumor resection was performed by two neurologists, A. Hughes Bennett and Rickman J. Godlee in 1884, London [1]. It resulted in the patient passing away 28 days afterward due to complications from the procedure. There are a variety of ways in which one can classify the different kinds of tumors. One such broad division can be made based on tumor malignancy characteristics; if the tumor is prone to encroaching on other areas of the body (i.e., malignant) or if it is non-cancerous (i.e., benign). Another method categorizes a tumor as per its origin, which can be termed as primary (i.e., originating in the brain or spinal cord) or secondary (i.e., originating from somewhere else in the body). We can further group them with primary brain tumors based on the type of cell causing the tumor mass. A glioma is a tumor that originates from glial cells and is known to be the most common form of malignant primary brain tumor. Some other kinds of primary tumors include meningiomas, ependymomas, and many types of lymphomas.

The patients who have undergone tumor resection surgery can suffer from deficits that can reduce their quality of life. Some of the common symptoms caused by motor cortex tumors include hemiparesis or hemiplegia, myopathy, ataxia, gait dysfunction, and spasticity. These symptoms justify the need for surgery to alleviate deficits and improve patients' quality of life if alternative therapeutic effects have failed. Furthermore, it also demonstrates the need for a safe resection where patients' odds of developing postoperative deficits are reduced. The intraoperative neurophysiological monitoring (IONM) of changes to the nervous system caused by surgical manipulations helps lower postoperative deficits and acts as an alarm system to warn and guide the surgeon. Cortical tumors surrounding the primary motor and premotor areas are likely to cause the symptoms above.

There are two approaches used in tumor resection, gross-total resection (GTR) and subtotal resection (STR). GTR involves the total removal of the tumor. It can be challenging to perform in cortical motor surgeries due to the necessity to differentiate between abnormal and healthy tissue. In contrast, STR calls for removing only the necessary parts of the tumor that can potentially alleviate the motor symptoms. Operating on the brain's motor regions becomes even more treacherous when considering how tumor masses may have distorted the anatomical landmarks that surgeons employ for resection surgeries. Thus, it is extremely crucial to use locating the functional anatomical regions such as the central sulcus, pre-central gyrus, post-central gyrus, and other functional brain regions surrounding the tumor. Knowledge about these alterations caused by tumors allows for safer surgical resections and guards the patients against potential damage to motor areas as protective actions would be taken.

IONM techniques can help identify and find the correct path of the central sulcus (CS) across both hemispheres while also mapping the cortical homunculus representation at the primary motor area. The method utilized to obtain such beneficial anatomical and functional knowledge during surgery is called motor mapping. Research had reported significant beneficial effects from motor mapping, such as the postoperative complication rate dropping from 21% to 13% when adequate neuro-monitoring was employed [2].

Fritsch and Hitzig (1870) pioneered the discovery of direct electrical cortical stimulation (DCS/DECS) of the animal brain [3]. Penfield and Boldrey demonstrated the mapping of the motor, sensory, and language cortices by directly stimulating an open cortex in human patients [4]. Different scientists have made tremendous progress throughout the 19th and 20th centuries to improve cortical motor mapping. George Ojemann introduced the Ojemann Cortical Stimulator (OCS), an electrical stimulator that improved Penfield's motor mapping technique. Taniguchi et al. proposed short multi-pulse stimulation using high frequencies during surgeries performed under general anesthesia [5]. In this technical report, we will discuss Penfield and Taniguchi's motor mapping methods with other considerations such as required tools, anesthetic recommendations, and modalities with their parametric values.

TECHNICAL REPORT

Preoperative evaluation of the patient

The human nervous system's physiological signals are unique to each individual, as the rest of the body's characteristics directly influences them. Unlike some static biological phenomena such as cardiac rhythms, brain physiology is highly dynamic, and it can change drastically during surgical procedures due to manipulations and surgical anesthesia. Hence, it is essential to establish the baseline for modalities such as somatosensory evoked potentials (SSEP) and motor evoked potentials (MEP). Cortical and sub-cortical motor mapping is needed for procedures including but not limited to brain tumors, intracranial aneurysms, arteriovenous malformation (AVM), and epilepsy surgeries. A multimodality approach is needed for the best postoperative outcome, including cortical sensory mapping with phase reversal, cortical motor mapping, subcortical motor mapping, electromyography (EMG), and electrocorticography (ECoG).

A detailed patient medical and surgical history should be taken and documented with any previous factors that may affect intraoperative cortical mapping data.

Anesthesia

The patient can be placed under general anesthesia for procedures that do not require evaluating the voluntary motor and language functions during surgery. When a patient's motor functions require multiple assessments or when language mapping is performed, awake craniotomy with the asleep-awake-asleep method of anesthesia must be employed. Hence, the patient will be placed under light anesthesia during the opening of the dura. After that, patients will be awakened for functional assessments during surgery. Baseline recordings will be helpful to account for the effect of anesthesia before surgical manipulation. Recommended anesthetic agents include a combination of propofol and an analgesic agent administered by the total intravenous anesthesia (TIVA) method. Other anesthetics that can be used include ketamine, etomidate, and benzodiazepines [6]. Dexmedetomidine, an alpha-adrenergic agonist, should be avoided due to its inhibitory effects on MEP [7]. Initially, inhalation anesthetics may be used for the patient's intubation, as significant TIVA transition will not affect recordings after incision [8]. However, inhalation anesthetics used for the entirety of the procedure can contribute to more postoperative deficits for patients, as thresholds for MEPs are higher in patients under inhalation anesthesia, leading to signals being weaker and more challenging to interpret. Also, it is essential to note that the stability of the patient's temperature is critical to consider at the site of recording as low temperatures increase signal latencies [6].

Intraoperative neurophysiological monitoring (IONM)

After the patient positioning on the operating table under anesthesia, subdermal needle electrodes are placed over the scalp as per the international 10-20 system for recording SSEP and EEG. Subdermal needle electrodes are placed in the face, upper and lower extremities muscles contralateral to the surgical site for recording EMG and MEP (Table 1). Surface adhesive electrodes are placed for stimulating peripheral (median, ulnar, posterior tibial, or femoral) nerves for SSEP and sensory mapping [8]. A phase reversal with sensory mapping is performed by placing a subdural grid or strip of the exposed cerebral cortex and stimulating the contralateral peripheral nerves. These grid electrodes are made of either stainless steel or platinum embedded in flexible silicone. Before performing the motor mapping, it is essential to localize the central sulcus (CS) correctly and to identify a potential shift in the sensory or motor cortices due to the physical expansion of the tumor mass. A 2 x 4 grid electrode is preferred for locating the CS, although other configurations are used as well, such as 1 x 6 or 1 x 8 electrode strips. Cortical grids or strips can be used for cortical stimulation in addition to the hand-held monopolar or bipolar probes (Figure 1).

Facial Muscles	Upper Extremities	Lower Extremities
Orbicularis Oculi	Deltoid	Quadriceps
Orbicularis Oris	Biceps Brachii	Tibialis Anterior
Tongue muscle	Flexor Carpi Ulnaris	Gastrocnemius
	Brachioradialis	Abductor Hallucis
	Abductor Pollicis Brevis	Extensor Hallucis Brevis
	Abductor Digiti Minimi	
	First Dorsal Interosseous	

Table 1: Electromyography. Recommended muscle recordings for electromyography (EMG) and direct electrical cortical stimulation (DECS), and subcortical stimulation.

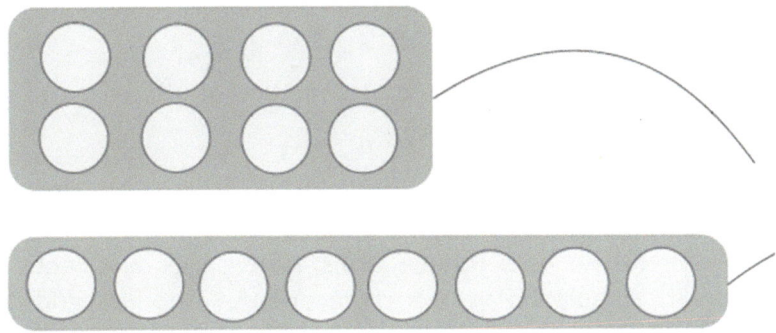

Figure 1: Subdural grids. Schematic presentation of the subdural cortical grids. A: Eight-contact grid (2 x 4); B: Eight-contact grid (1 x 8).

Two techniques, Penfield, and Taniguchi, have evolved for intraoperative cortical and subcortical mapping of the corticospinal tracts. Either of these two methods can be utilized based on tumor location, patient history, surgical procedure, and other factors.

A) Penfield cortical (50-Hz) technique

A distinguished neurosurgeon, Dr. Wilder Penfield, first described this technique in 1937. This technique is accomplished with a hand-held bipolar stimulator using a 50-Hz stimulation (interstimulus interval of 20 milliseconds) with a train of monophasic cathodal pulses of an individual pulse width of 0.5 milliseconds [4]. The stimulation is applied to the cortex for a duration of 2 to 5 seconds, with a 5-10 seconds interval between each stimulus (Figure 2). Each stimulation point should not be stimulated consecutively. Direct cortical stimulation is performed at a lower intensity to the exposed cortex, starting from 2.0 milliamperes (mA). The stimulus should be increased in increments until either a positive response, maximum allowable stimulation of 20 mA is reached, or if after discharges (AD) are seen in ECoG recordings. If ADs are present, iced cold saline solution (4°C) should be quickly applied to the exposed stimulated cortex.

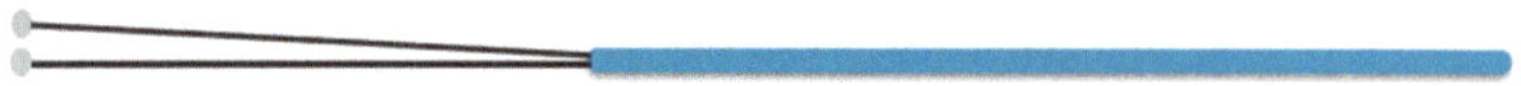

Figure 2: Bipolar probe. Schematic presentation of a bipolar ball tip hand-held probe.

Cortical areas of the face, tongue, arms, hands, legs, and feet are identified with stimulation and muscle recording. A subdural grid can also be placed over the area to monitor the status of the patient's motor function and to alert the surgeon of any changes that might later incur deficits for the patient [4]. Recording and stimulation parameters suggested for the Penfield method are specified in Table 2 and Table 3, respectively.

Recording Parameters		
Specification	Penfield	Taniguchi
Low-cut filter	10 Hz	10 Hz
High-cut filter	5000 Hz	5000 Hz
Notch Filter	Off	Off
Dynamic Range (Input Gain)	200-500 µV/div	200-500 µV/div
Sensitivity	200 µV	200 µV
Time-base	100 ms/div	10 ms/div
Electrode impedance	> 5 kΩ	> 5 kΩ

Table 2: Recording parameters.

Recording parameters suggested by Penfield and Taniguchi. Hz = Hertz, µs = microseconds, µV = microvolts, div = division, ms = milliseconds, kΩ = kiloohms.

Stimulation Parameters		
Specification	Penfield	Taniguchi
Type of Stimulator	Bipolar	Monopolar
Type of Pulse (Phase)	Biphasic or Monophasic	Monophasic Anodal
Frequency	50 Hz	250-500 Hz
Pulse width	300 - 1000 μs	500 μs
Intensity	2 - 20 mA	2 - 20 mA
Duration of stimulation	2 - 5 s	20 μs

Table 3: Stimulation parameters.

Recommended stimulation parameters for Penfield and Taniguchi. Hz = Hertz, μs = microseconds, mA = milliamperes, s = seconds, ms = milliseconds.

B) Taniguchi cortical technique

In 1993, Taniguchi first published a high-frequency multi-pulse short train technique for direct cortical motor mapping. A hand-held monopolar ball tip stimulator can be used to stimulate the motor cortex during the surgery to determine the motor fibers' status at risk (Figure 3). This method uses a higher frequency of stimulation to the motor cortex at a rate of 250 to 500 Hz [4]. Electromyography (EMG) is used to record myogenic responses from the contralateral target muscles. This method provides the ability to monitor corticospinal tracts' functional integrity throughout the procedure and alert the surgeon for any potential damage to the functional brain areas. Thus, it can help determine if further tumor resection can be continued or not (Figures 4-6). Recording and stimulation parameters suggested for the Taniguchi method are specified in Table 2 and Table 3, respectively.

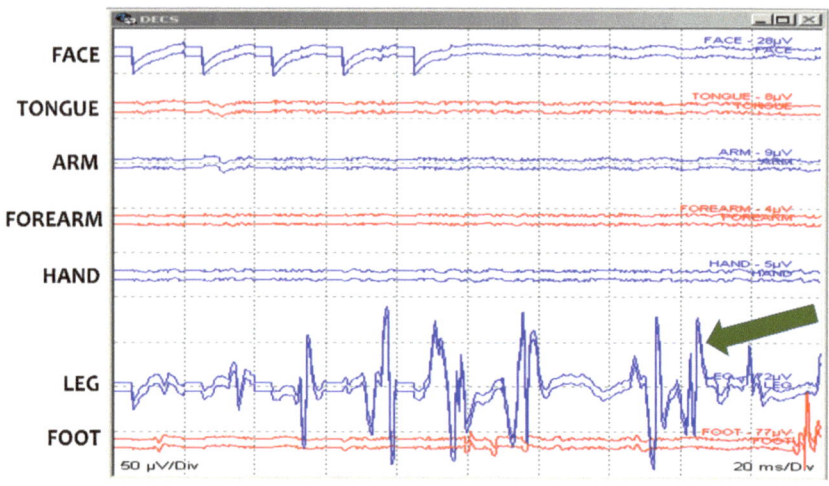

Figure 3: Motor mapping: Penfield method.

Motor mapping responses after bipolar hand-held stimulation using a Penfield 50 Hz method. Multiple responses are present in leg muscles (green arrow). Face (Orbicularis Oris), Tongue, Arm (Deltoid/Biceps Brachii), Forearm (Brachioradialis/Flexor Carpi Ulnaris), Hand (Abductor Pollicis Brevis/Abductor digiti minimi), Leg (Tibialis Anterior), and Foot (Abductor Hallucis) muscles.

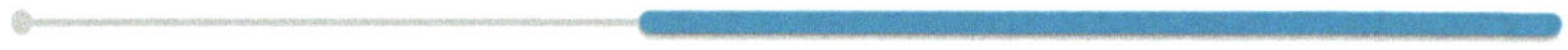

Figure 4: Monopolar probe. Schematic presentation of a hand-held ball tip monopolar probe.

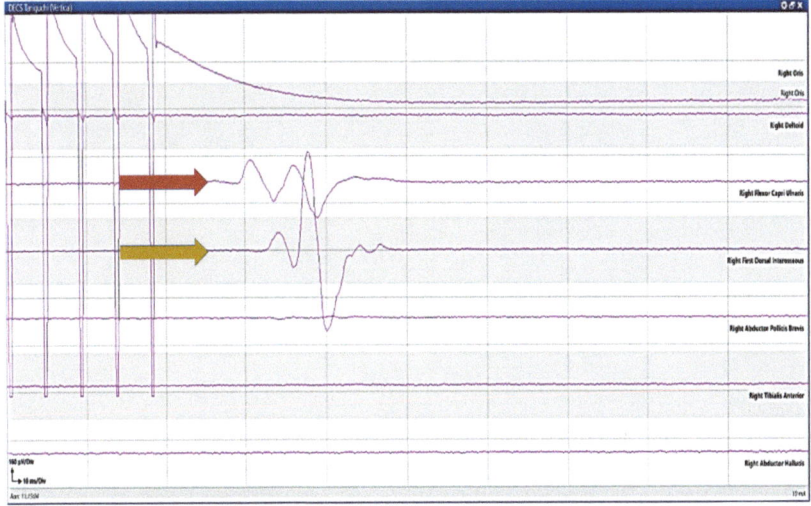

Figure 5: Motor mapping: Taniguchi method. Motor mapping responses after monopolar hand-held stimulation using a Taniguchi high-frequency method. Motor evoked responses are present in the right Flexor Carpi Ulnaris (red arrow) and First Dorsal Interosseous (orange arrow) muscles.

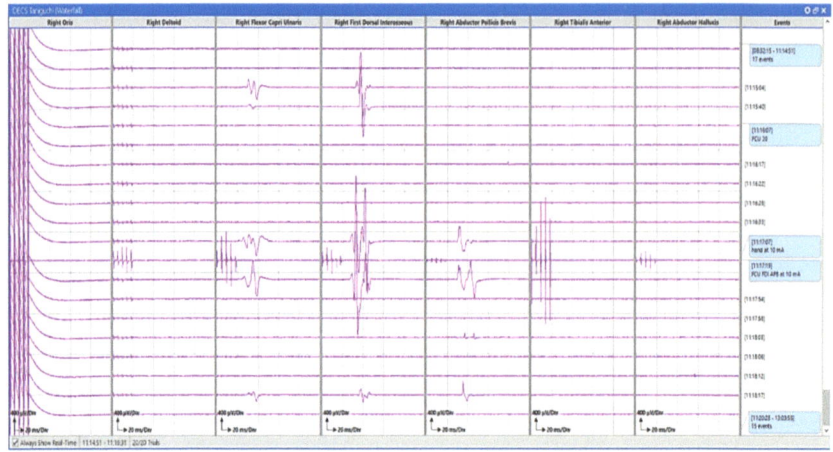

Figure 6: Motor mapping stack: Taniguchi method. Motor mapping responses in stack view after monopolar hand-held stimulation using a Taniguchi high-frequency method. Motor evoked responses are stacked in the right Flexor Carpi Ulnaris, First Dorsal Interosseous, and Abductor Pollicis Brevis muscles.

Sub-cortical mapping

Sub-cortical motor mapping is used for tumors that are near or within the corticospinal tract (CST). A monopolar ball tip electrode is used in conjunction with the suction device used for tumor resection [9]. The subcortical CST fibers are identified by stimulation and recording the motor thresholds (MT), which act as an indicator of how far away from the CST the resection has taken place. MTs are measured in milliamps (mA), and every 1.0 mA change reflects a 1-mm distance change from the CST [9, 10]. The surgeon will continue to proceed until an MT of 7 mA is seen. Once MT of 7 mA is identified, it is generally recommended that the surgeon stops the resection of the tumor. Proceeding past 7 mA will stimulate the CST and will produce MEPs, and resection of tissue past this point increases the likelihood of having postoperative motor deficits in the patient [10]. Szelényi et al.

showed that monopolar cathodal stimulation is more effective than the bipolar cathodal stimulus for eliciting MEPs for sub-cortical mapping (Table 4) [11].

Sub-cortical Stimulation Parameters	
Intensity	2 - 20 mA
Type of stimulation	Monopolar Cathodal
Duration of pulse	0.5 - 1 ms
Frequency	250 - 500 Hz
Number of Pulses	4 - 5
Interstimulus Interval	3 - 4 ms

Table 4: Sub-cortical stimulation.

Sub-cortical mapping stimulation parameters. mA = milliamperes, ms = milliseconds, Hz = Hertz.

Electromyography (EMG)

Spontaneous electromyography (sEMG) signals from the contralateral face, upper and lower extremity muscles should be continuously recorded and monitored during the surgery [8]. EMG provides real-time feedback about any changes in muscle activity (Tables 1, 2).

Electroencephalography (EEG)

Electroencephalography (EEG) is a spontaneous recording of the cerebral cortex's electrical activity recorded from the scalp. Scalp EEG consists of the summation of excitatory and inhibitory postsynaptic potentials of cortical pyramidal neurons. EEG is utilized to monitor brain perfusion as well as the depth of anesthesia [8]. If burst suppression is noted, it needs to be addressed immediately to provide accurate neuromonitoring. It is important to maintain a consistent depth of anesthesia using spontaneous and processed EEG. This will allow us to avoid any variability in stimulation thresholds and accurate intraoperative cortical and subcortical stimulation (Table 5).

EEG Recording Parameters	
Parameter	Value
Low-cut filter	1 Hz
High-cut filter	70 Hz
Notch filter	50 Hz (Europe/Asia) or 60 Hz (USA)
Dynamic Range (Input Gain)	30 µV/div
Sensitivity	70 µV/div
Sweep	1000 ms/div
Electrode impedance	> 5 kΩ

Table 5: Electroencephalography. Electroencephalography (EEG) recording parameters. Hz = Hertz, ms = milliseconds, µV = microvolts, div = division, kΩ = kiloohms.

Electrocorticography (ECoG)

Electrocorticography (ECoG) is recorded intraoperatively by placing subdural grid electrodes and strips directly on the brain surface under the dura (Table 6). The spatial and temporal resolution of ECoG is higher than scalp EEG with no attenuation of the signal by the scalp and the skull. Therefore, the signal-to-noise ratio of ECoG is significantly better than scalp EEG. As compared to the scalp EEG, the ECoG waveforms are typically higher amplitude, higher frequencies, and can see dipole sources of both interictal and ictal activity. The subdural grids and strips electrodes are placed temporarily during the surgery to localize any epileptiform discharges (or after-discharges) during direct cortical stimulation (Figure 7). ECoG is also used to map and resect any epileptogenic regions of the brain (Figure 8). ECoG should be performed along with DECS for active tracking of after-discharges and preventing any seizure by immediately applying ice saline solution (4°C) to the exposed cortex.

ECoG Recording Parameters	
Parameter	Value
Low-cut filter	1 Hz
High-cut filter	70 Hz
Notch filter	Off
Dynamic Range (Input Gain)	20 µV/div
Sensitivity	100 µV/div
Sweep	500 ms/div
Electrode impedance	> 5 kΩ

Table 6: Electrocorticography. Electrocorticography (ECoG) recording parameters. Hz = Hertz, µV = microvolts, div = division, ms = milliseconds, kΩ = kiloohms.

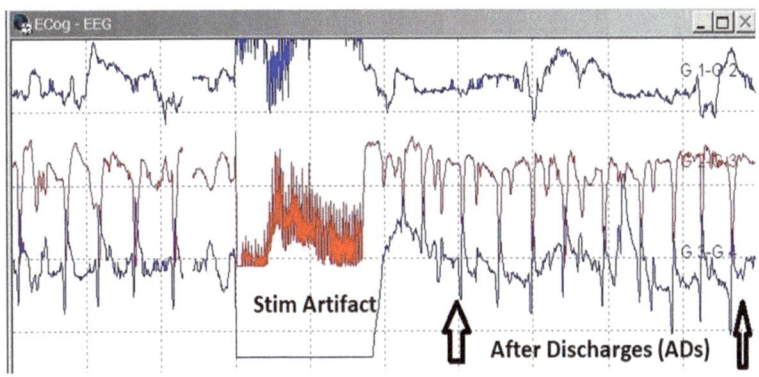

Figure 7: Electrocorticography. Electrocorticography (ECoG) recordings are showing stimulation artifact induced after discharges (white arrows).

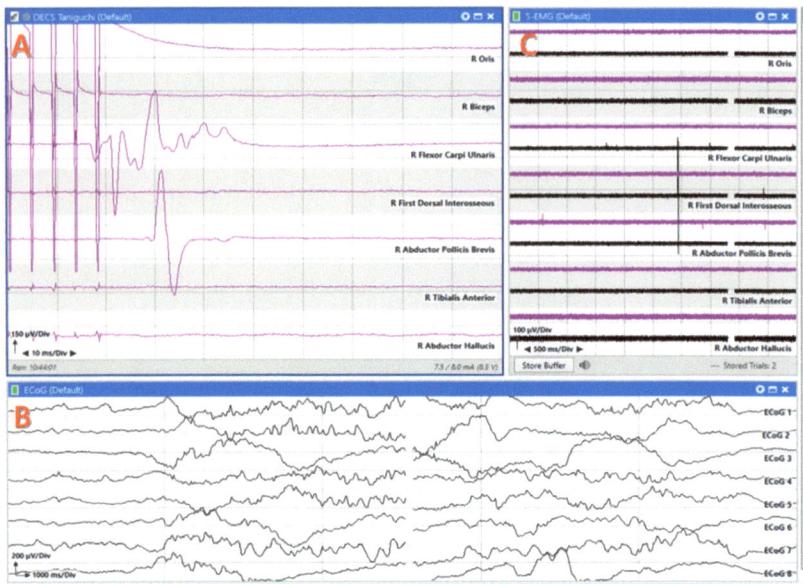

Figure 8: Multimodality mapping. Multimodality motor mapping with responses after monopolar hand-held stimulation using a Taniguchi high-frequency method. A: Motor evoked responses are present in the right Flexor Carpi Ulnaris and Abductor Pollicis Brevis muscles. B: Electrocorticography (ECoG), and C: Electromyography (EMG).

Train of four (TOF)

Train of four (TOF) is an additional important modality for consideration during motor mapping procedures involving the application of muscle relaxants. TOF is used to assess the level of the neuromuscular junction blockage due to muscle relaxants. Four pulses of stimulation per train are needed to facilitate response in selected peripheral nerves. The stimulation parameters are intensity between 10 and 100 mA, with a frequency of 2 Hz, pulse-width of 200 μs, stimulation duration of 2 seconds, an interstimulus interval of 0.5 ms an inter-train interval of 10 seconds [12]. The recording parameter includes a sweep of 20 ms/div, with a gain of 100-500 μV/div (Table 7).

TOF Responses Present of Four Twitches	Degree of Neuromuscular Blockage
4 out of 4 responses	0 – 5%
3 out of 4 responses	65 – 75%
2 out of 4 responses	85%
1 out of 4 responses	95%
0 out of 4 responses	100%

Table 7: Train of four.

Train of four (TOF) responses are representing the level of neuromuscular blockade during surgical anesthesia.

Postoperative evaluation of the patient

The patient should undergo evaluation based on the Medical Research Council (MRC) Scale score (M1 to M5), National Institutes of Health Stroke Scale score, and Karnofsky Performance Scale score. The patient needs to be evaluated for postoperative deficits immediately following surgery. We recommend that postoperative evaluations be performed after 24 hours, 48 hours, two weeks, three months, and six months after the procedure.

DISCUSSION

The experience of the technologist and neurophysiologist is an essential factor for accurate motor mapping of the brain. Higher knowledge, experience, and comprehensive experience of the neurophysiological monitoring teams improve their ability to detect and preempt complications during the surgery [13].

According to Krieg et al., many cases of false negatives (4.5%) arise from ischemic or hemorrhaging events that occur postoperatively [14]. They are not false negatives from monitoring but instead result from accumulated damage to blood vessels during surgery that manifests after the neuromonitoring has concluded. Adequate training, proper equipment, and instruments are vital towards mitigating the risk of mistakes [6]. False positives are also critical as they impede surgical progress and foster distrust in the surgeon towards future alerts. Potentially, it leads to the loss of MEPs where proper care could have been taken to avoid such incidents [6]. Wrong interpretations also play their part in getting false results. It is highly recommended to use the predefined and well-established criteria provided by research and guidelines based on types of surgeries. Some of the alert criteria include the threshold of stimulation criteria, amplitude criteria, and morphology criteria [15-17]. Cedzich et al. corroborated the idea of employing EMG as a measure of intact motor pathways and mapping the cortex region, as it would not need the higher stimulation that inherently produces the risk of invoking seizure activity [18]. Also, the need have to see limb movements to confirm the intact MEPs can be avoidable, especially for the microsurgical interventions. EMG allows for lower direct cortical stimulation to verify functional integrity.

Testing motor function via stimulating the motor strip under general anesthesia with the application of a bipolar stimulator was first employed by Fritsch and Hitzig. It is beneficial for motor mapping in cortical and sub-cortical regions, with better spatial stimulation resolution when compared to monopolar stimulation. However, it has been demonstrated that monopolar stimulation requires less amplitude for stimulation as it can directly activate pyramidal axons and induce repetitive excitation of the corticospinal tract (CST) while reducing the chance of damaging neural tissue [19].

CONCLUSIONS

Intraoperative electrical stimulation of the corticospinal tract (CST) can be performed by two techniques, 50 Hz frequency Penfield and the high-frequency multi-pulse Taniguchi methods. Both methods provide a safe, helpful, and reliable resection near the central sulcus. A multimodality approach with sensory mapping, direct electrical cortical stimulation (DECS), electromyography (EMG), and electrocorticography (ECoG) increases the mapping accuracy at the lowest threshold with minimal risk of intraoperative seizures. Mapping of the motor cortex should be done after identifying the central sulcus with sensory mapping. DECS should be performed simultaneously with spontaneous EMG and ECoG to identify the ADs before the onset of seizures.

This review illustrates the technical details involved in intraoperative cortical motor mapping during brain surgeries. Following a set of standardized guidelines and taking steps with a clear and concise methodology inside the operating room helps patients come out of critical surgical interventions with minimal neurological deficits. The viability of employing advanced intraoperative neurophysiological monitoring techniques helps in guiding the surgeon with confidence and clarity. Involving the teams with experience in surgical procedures and IONM will have a better patient outcome as compared to less or non-experienced members. We propose that a multimodality approach towards neuromonitoring is necessary to minimize the probability of postoperative complications.

DISCLOSURES

Human subjects: Consent was obtained by all participants in this study. **Animal subjects:** All authors have confirmed that this study did not involve animal subjects or tissue. **Conflicts of interest:** In compliance with the ICMJE uniform disclosure form, all authors declare the following: **Payment/services info:** All authors have declared that no financial support was received from any organization for the submitted work. **Financial relationships:** All authors have declared that they have no financial relationships at present or within the previous three years with any organizations that might have an interest in the submitted work. **Other relationships:** All authors have declared that there are no other relationships or activities that could appear to have influenced the submitted work.

REFERENCES

1. Kirkpatrick DB: The first primary brain-tumor operation. J Neurosurg. 1984, 61:809-813. 10.3171/jns.1984.61.5.0809

2. Gerritsen JKW, Arends L, Klimek M, Dirven CMF, Edouard Vincent AJP: Impact of intraoperative stimulation mapping on high-grade glioma surgery outcome: a meta-analysis. Acta Neurochir. 2019, 161:99-107. 10.1007/s00701-018-3732-4

3. Carlson C, Devinsky O: The excitable cerebral cortex. Fritsch G, Hitzig E. Über die elektrische Erregbarkeit des Grosshirns. Arch Anat Physiol Wissen 1870; 37: 300-32. Epilepsy Behav. 2009, 15:131-132. 10.1016/j.yebeh.2009.03.002

4. Penfield W, Boldrey E: Somatic motor and sensory representation in the cerebral cortex of man as studied by electrical stimulation. Brain. 1937, 60:389-443. 10.1093/brain/60.4.389

5. Taniguchi M, Cedzich C, Schramm J, Cedzich C, Schramm J: Modification of cortical stimulation for motor evoked potentials under general anesthesia: technical description. Neurosurgery. 1993, 32:219-226. 10.1227/00006123-199302000-00011

6. MacDonald DB, Skinner S, Shils J, Yingling C: Intraoperative motor evoked potential monitoring - A position statement by the American Society of Neurophysiological Monitoring. Clin Neurophysiol. 2013, 124:2291-2316. 10.1016/j.clinph.2013.07.025

7. Mahmoud M, Sadhasivam S, Salisbury S, et al.: Susceptibility of transcranial electric motor-evoked potentials to varying targeted blood levels of dexmedetomidine during spine surgery. Anesthesiology. 2010, 112:1364-1373. 10.1097/ALN.0b013e3181d74f55

8. Jahangiri FR: Surgical Neurophysiology: A Reference Guide to Intraoperative Neurophysiological Monitoring (IONM), 2nd Ed. CreateSpace, 2012.

9. Raabe A, Beck J, Schucht P, Seidel K: Continuous dynamic mapping of the corticospinal tract during surgery of motor eloquent brain tumors: evaluation of a new method. J Neurosurg. 2014, 120:1015-1024. 10.3171/2014.1.JNS13909

10. Schucht P, Seidel K, Murek M, et al.: Low-threshold monopolar motor mapping for resection of lesions in motor eloquent areas in children and adolescents. J Neurosurg Pediatr. 2014, 13:572-578. 10.3171/2014.1.PEDS13369

11. Szelényi A, Senft C, Jardan M, Forster MT, Franz K, Seifert V, Vatter H: Intra-operative subcortical electrical stimulation: a comparison of two methods. Clin Neurophysiol. 2011, 122:1470-1475. 10.1016/j.clinph.2010.12.055

12. McGrath CD, Hunter JM: Monitoring of neuromuscular block. Contin Educ Anaesth Crit Care Pain. 2006, 6:7-12. 10.1093/bjaceaccp/mki067

13. Kim SM, Kim SH, Seo DW, Lee KW: Intraoperative neurophysiologic monitoring: basic principles and recent update. J Korean Med Sci. 2013, 28:1261-1269. 10.3346/jkms.2013.28.9.1261

14. Krieg SM, Shiban E, Droese D, et al.: Predictive value and safety of intraoperative neurophysiological monitoring with motor evoked potentials in glioma surgery. Neurosurgery. 2012, 70:1060-1070. 10.1227/NEU.0b013e31823f5ade

15. Nuwer MR, Emerson RG, Galloway FG, et al.: Evidence-based guideline update: intraoperative spinal monitoring with somatosensory and transcranial electrical motor evoked potentials. J Clin Neurophysiol. 2012, 29:101-108. 10.1097/WNP.0b013e31824a397e

16. Calancie B, Harris W, Broton JG, Alexeeva N, Green BA: "Threshold-level" multi-pulse transcranial electrical stimulation of motor cortex for intraoperative monitoring of spinal motor tracts: description of method and comparison to somatosensory evoked potential monitoring. J Neurosurg. 1998, 88:457-470. 10.3171/jns.1998.88.3.0457.

17. Quiñones-Hinojosa A, Lyon R, Zada G, et al.: Changes in transcranial motor evoked potentials during intramedullary spinal cord tumor resection correlate with postoperative motor function. Neurosurgery. 2005, 56:982-993. 10.1227/01.NEU.0000158203.29369.37

18. Cedzich C, Taniguchi M, Schäfer S, Schramm J: Somatosensory evoked potential phase reversal and direct motor cortex stimulation during surgery in and around the central region. Neurosurgery. 1996, 38:962-970. 10.1097/00006123-199605000-00023

19. Kombos T, Suess O, Funk T, Kern BC, Brock M: Intra-operative mapping of the motor cortex during surgery in and around the motor cortex. Acta Neurochirurgica. 2000, 142:263-268. 10.1007/s007010050034.

Citation:

Jahangiri FR, Dobariya A, Kruse A, Kalyta O, Moorman JD. Mapping of the Motor Cortex. Cureus. 2020 Sep 25;12(9):e10645. doi: 10.7759/cureus.10645. PMID: 33133815; PMCID: PMC7586383.

MAPPING OF THE BRAIN

CHAPTER 3

MAPPING OF THE LANGUAGE CORTEX

Faisal R. Jahangiri[1,2,3], Gurtegh S. Chima[1], Martha Pearson[1], Jacob Jackson[1], Arshad A. Siddiqui[3]

[1]Department of Applied Cognition and Neuroscience, The University of Texas at Dallas, Richardson, TX; [2]Axis Neuromonitoring LLC, Richardson, TX; [3]Dept. of Neurosurgery, Neuroscience Institute, Hamad Medica Corporation, Doha, Qatar.

ABSTRACT

Awake craniotomy with Intraoperative Neurophysiological Language Mapping (INLM) is an established procedure for patients undergoing surgery to resection tumors in the language cortex area. INLM and continuous neurophysiological monitoring allow assessment of the language function, which is not possible under general anesthesia. INLM of the eloquent brain areas provides a helpful tool to the operating surgeon in reducing the risks associated with tumor resection in the motor and language cortex. We present a literature review and the technical method used for INLM by utilizing direct electrical cortical stimulation. We also report the usefulness of INLM for evaluation of the language function during resection of cortical tumors, epilepsy foci, and arteriovenous malformations (AVMs) located near language areas. First, the central sulcus is identified by sensory mapping, followed by the motor cortex's identification by Direct Electrical Cortical Stimulation (DECS). Neurological assessment of the patient is done by auditory and visual feedback. The patient is asked to repeat numbers, days, words, sentences, read words, and name pictures during cortical stimulation. DECS may cause a slurring or speech arrest. Electrocorticography (ECoG) is also performed during cortical stimulation to identify any after-discharges. The patients are examined immediately postoperatively, 24 hours, after one week, six months, and 12 months. Bipolar DECS for motor mapping with ECoG can safely and reliably be utilized to identify essential language areas with minimizing permanent language deficits and maximize the extent of tumor resection.

Keywords: Language mapping, Broca's, Wernicke's, tumors, eloquent area.

INTRODUCTION

A neurosurgical procedure such as an awake craniotomy for resection of epileptic foci or gliomas is safely used near the brain's language areas. In the 1860s, the language areas of the brain were identified by Broca and Wernicke. Later in 1886, Sir Victor Horsley identified an epileptic focus by electrical stimulation of the cortex in an awake surgery. In the 1940s-50s, an American-Canadian neurosurgeon Wilder G. Penfield performed and published mapping of the brain with electrical stimulation response during awake epilepsy surgery. The Neurolept Anesthesia (NLA) was introduced in the 1960s, which allowed surgery in awake patients without any tracheal intubation. After the introduction of intravenous anesthesia using propofol in the 1990s, awake craniotomy with functional brain mapping with electrical stimulation became more common.

The mapping of the language areas helps in preventing permanent postoperative dysfunction by preserving these language areas. Presently, researchers are attempting to fully explore and standardize the areas responsible for language-eloquence to decrease the likelihood of injury during tumor removal and epilepsy surgeries. Emerging technologies such as functional imaging of the brain and intraoperative neuronavigation and functional brain mapping with electrical stimulation under an awake state may facilitate a more significant expansion of resection area while feasibly minimizing risk and the associated morbidity profile [1].

Surgical resection near the cortical language area involves a risk of permanent changes to the recovering patients' lifestyle. Long-term deficits in verbal/linguistic ability and perceptual lifestyle changes can be observed, where social exchange behavior is greatly limited by the intended but unguided surgical procedure.

TECHNICAL REPORT

Preoperative Assessment

Functional magnetic resonance imaging (fMRI) can help identify various brain areas by activating them during a particular mental process. Diffusion tensor imaging (DTI) can identify the white matter fibers traveling as bundles or tracts (tractography). In 1948, Jun Wada developed the Wada test, which is considered the gold standard test for identifying the cerebral hemisphere dominant for the language area.

On the day of the surgery, preoperative language testing of the patient is performed. The patient's baseline language status is identified preoperatively and used as a reference during the surgery through language mapping (Tables 1 and 2). Preoperative language testing can be primarily to familiarize the patient with the test style. This mitigates any discrepancies in the patients' performance during the surgery, limiting the possible occurrence of an error during the intraoperative awake testing without appropriate stimulation of the cortex's areas. Test battery must be given before the surgery, before anesthesia, and then once again, during the surgery (Table 3).

Language Region	Sub-Region	Function	Associated Deficits/Aphasias	Tasks used to identify aphasias	Possible significant events	Possible error (false localizations)
Broca's Area (BA)	Pars Opercularis	Speech production, commonly used preposition & word generation	Speech arrest, failure to produce words, hesitation, slurring	Rote tasks (counting, alphabet, days of the week, months of the year), preposition task	Arrest, failure to produce words, hesitation slurring, incorrect/nonsense words, perseveration	Activation of face motor area interpreted as BA
	Pars Triangularis	Speech production	Loss/difficulty producing language	Rote tasks (counting, alphabet, days of the week, months of the year), noun & verb production task	Slowing, slurring, hesitation, arrest	Activation of face motor area interpreted as BA, missing hints, word category errors
	Pre-Frontal Cortex (Pars Orbitalis)	Word production & development (nouns/verbs)	Inability to produce language, failure to carry complex & simple conversation	Repeating (words, sentences), noun & verb production task	Slowing, slurring, hesitation, arrest, literal & verbal paraphrasing errors, nonsense words	Activation of face motor area interpreted as BA

Table 1: Broca's Area (BA). Broca's language area, its sub-regions, function, associated deficits, tasks used to identify aphasias, possible significant events, and potential errors during language mapping

Language Region	Sub-Region	Function	Associated Deficits/Aphasias	Tasks used to identify aphasias	Possible significant events	Possible error (false localizations)
Wernicke's Area (WA)	Superior Temporal Gyrus (STG)	Language comprehension (with primary auditory input)	Loss/difficulty understanding language, anomia	Sentence Completion (SC), Phrase Repetition (PR), ON	Error in the selection, patient not understanding, need a question repeated, random word phrase generation, literal/verbal aphasia	Passing off a subtle language event as an environmental issue (patient having trouble hearing)
	Angular Gyrus (AG)	Receives visual input related to language comprehension/reading	Primarily visual-based language deficits (reading)	Word/sentence reading, ON in adjunct with the above	The patient having trouble visualizing words/sentences, literal/verbal aphasia, paraphasias, hesitation	Passing off a subtle language event as an environmental issue (assuming problem are a result of anesthesia/exhaustion)
	Supramarginal Gyrus (SMG)	Process visual/auditory receptive language projects to frontal language areas	Difficulty/inability to comprehend speech, including morphological errors, literal/verbal paraphasic errors. Neologisms, acalculia	DECS disruption	N/A	Misrepresenting visual language deficits as an inability to see presentation stimuli
Inferior Temporal Language Area (ITLA)	N/A	Primarily ON	Anomia	ON	Inability to name objects	Inability to name objects
Arcuate Fibers	N/A	Linking WA with BA language areas	Conductive aphasia, fragmented/broken speech, inarticulate	Combination of Repetition, word generation, SC	N/A	N/A

Table 2: Wernicke's Area (WA). Wernicke's language area, its sub-regions, function, associated deficits, tasks used to identify aphasias, possible significant events, and potential errors during language mapping.

Anesthesia

The Asleep-awake-asleep cycle is used for craniotomy procedures with language mapping [2,3]. The patient is intubated with total intravenous anesthesia (TIVA) using propofol (or sodium pentothal). Mayfield stabilizes the patient's head with implanted pins. Hyperventilation is performed before opening the dura. The patient is extubated and awaken for mapping of the language areas. Once the mapping and the surgical procedure are complete, the patient is intubated with a fiberoptic laryngoscope for general anesthesia.

Alternately, during the conscious sedation protocol, the sedation is initiated and maintained with propofol or midazolam and/or dexmedetomidine. Fentanyl or sufentanil is used for analgesia. The infusion is typically stopped 10-15 minutes before the mapping. The patient is awake for mapping during the critical parts of resection during the surgery. Once the resection is complete, the propofol is started again.

Intraoperative Neurophysiological Language Mapping (INLM)

After patient sedation, the patient is positioned in the supine position with his head affixed to the three-pin Mayfield frame. The stimulation surface adhesive electrodes for median nerve Somatosensory Evoked Potentials (SSEP) are placed on the wrists bilaterally. Subdermal needle electrodes for Electromyography (EMG) recordings are placed in the contralateral face, upper, and lower extremity muscles. Subdermal needle electrodes are also placed on the scalp for SSEP and Electroencephalogram (EEG) recordings. Baseline median nerve SSEP responses are recorded bilaterally along with the baseline scalp EEG [4].

The stereotactic navigational system is then registered and used to make an appropriate skin incision. The head is prepped using betadine and alcohol solutions. A local anesthetic is injected into the dermis. A skin incision is made. The skull surface overlying the tumor is exposed, and the stereotactic system is used to identify the tumor margins. A standard craniotomy is performed.

Awake craniotomies are used frequently in contemporary neurosurgery due to low failure rates, with failure constituting both expressive and perceptive linguistic limitations in the patient postoperatively. While various protocols exist to map language areas during these operations, we will outline the process to provide a guide for effective operational analysis of linguistic centers for brain tissue excision surgery. While the patient is awake, the test battery is again repeated, with the surgeon using the following procedure for testing the cortex and simultaneously referencing the patient's task performance (Table 3).

Craniotomy should expose a tumor (or implicated epileptogenic tissues) and 3 cm of the surrounding brain surface. A hand-held one-millimeter bipolar probe positioned 5.0 mm apart is used for direct cortical stimulation. A biphasic square-wave pulse of 200-500 microseconds (μs) pulse width, trains of 50 or 60 Hertz (Hz), starting with a low stimulus constant current at 1.5-mA and increased to a maximum of 20 mA or identification of After Discharges (ADs). However, a square-wave pulse under 7.0 mA is preferred. The cortex is mapped every 5–10 mm, and positive stimulation sites at which language impairment was caused (by the process of awake craniotomy testing) are marked with sterile numbered tickets [1]. The cortex is then excised/lesioned with minimal damage done to cortical tissues responsible for successful communication when deep anesthesia is resumed. The surgery can then conclude with the surgeon completing the procedure.

Sensory Mapping:

Following adequate exposure of the cortex, a six-grid (1 x 6) or eight-grid (1x8 or 2x4) subdural electrode is placed on the cortical surface over the area of the presumed central sulcus (CS) for waveform interpretation in all four planes, anterior-posterior and medial-lateral. Contralateral median nerve stimulation is used to generate phase reversal at the central sulcus (Fig 1). Recording filters are set at 30-3000Hz with a time base of 100 milliseconds [5]. The CS and somatosensory cortex are localized by generating multiple sensory maps by stimulating the contralateral median nerve at a current of 20-35 mA between frequencies of 2.66-4.79 Hz. Mapping continued until the triphasic waveform was generated with a P25 peak directly over the central sulcus and part of the P20/N30-N20/P30 complex (Fig 2).

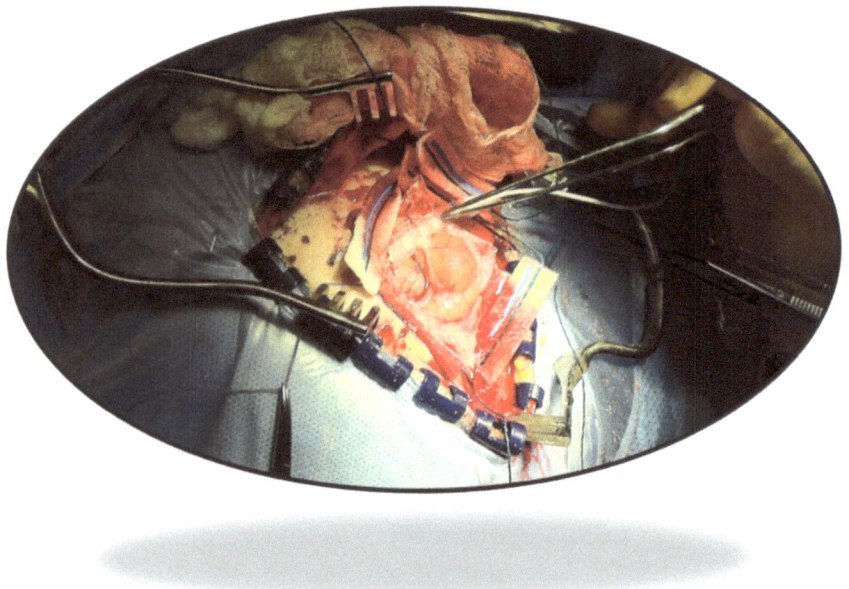

Figure 1: Cortical grid. Placement of a cortical grid (six contact 1x6) over the exposed area for sensory mapping phase reversal.

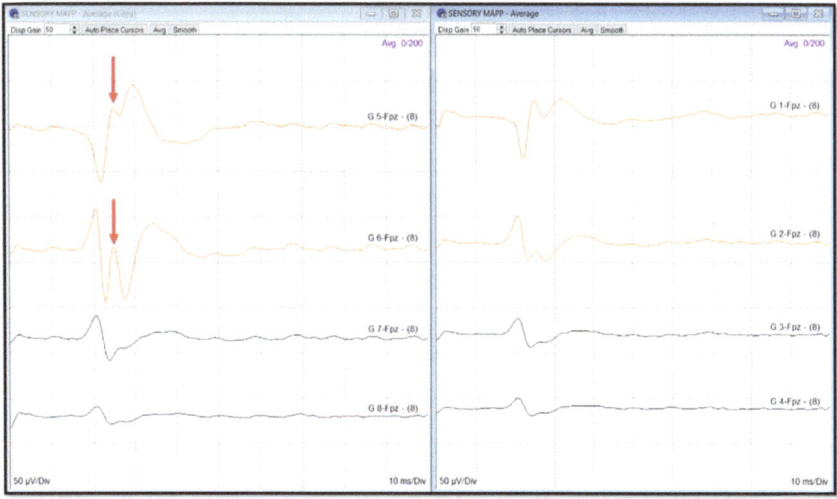

Figure 2: Cortical Sensory Mapping. Sensory mapping phase reversal. On-axis median nerve sensory mapping by a 2x4 grid with a triphasic phase reversal, including a P25 response. The phase reversal is between G1/2 and G5/6. The responses from G1 and G2 are pre-central, and G2, G3, G4, G6, G7, and G8 are post-central.

Motor mapping (By Direct Electrical Cortical Stimulation - DECS):

After localization of the central sulcus, motor mapping is performed by cortical motor mapping using Direct Electrical Cortical Stimulation (DECS) and Electrocorticography (ECoG). DECS can be done by two methods [6]. The high-frequency short pulse Taniguchi method is performed by using a monopolar anodal hand-held ball tip probe with a pulse duration of 500 μs, 4 or 5 pulses at a frequency of 250-500 Hz. The stimulation intensity is applied between 2-30 mA. The slow frequency long pulse Penfield method is performed by using hand-held bipolar ball tips probe with a pulse duration of 300-500 microseconds at a frequency of 50 Hz. Stimulation is applied for three to five seconds at each site. During the stimulus, the subdural grid electrodes are placed on the exposed cortex close to the stimulation sites to monitor ECoG for the presence of ADs or seizure activity. The stimulation is initiated at an intensity of 2.0 mA and increased as needed until a positive response (Compound Muscle Action Potential- CAMP) or After Discharges (ADs) is elicited, or until clinical seizure activity is encountered (with a maximum limit of 20 milliamperes/mA) (Fig 3).

There are two types of responses to electrical stimulation of the brain. When the response is induced, it is known as a "positive mapping," When the response is suppressed, it is known as "negative mapping."

Stimulation Parameters		
Specification	Penfield	Taniguchi
Type of Stimulator	Bipolar	Monopolar
Type of Pulse (Phase)	Biphasic or Monophasic	Monophasic
Frequency	50 Hz	250-500 Hz
Pulse width	300 – 1000 μs	500 μs
Intensity	2 – 10 mA	2 – 20 mA
Duration of stimulation	2 – 5 s	10 – 20 ms

Table 3: Stimulation Parameters. Penfield and Taniguchi's methods suggested stimulation parameters. (Hertz=Hz, microseconds=μs, milliseconds=ms, milliamperes=mA, seconds=s).

MAPPING OF THE BRAIN

Recording Parameters		
Specification	Penfield	Taniguchi
Low-cut filter	10 Hz	10 Hz
High-cut filter	5000 Hz	5000 Hz
Notch Filter	60 Hz (Off for ECoG)	50 Hz or 60 Hz
Gain	200	200-500
Sensitivity	200 µV	200 µV
Time-base	100 ms/div	100 ms/div

Table 4: Recording Parameters. Recording parameters suggested by Penfield and Taniguchi. (Hertz=Hz, microvolts=µV, milliseconds=ms, divison=div, Electrocortocography=ECoG).

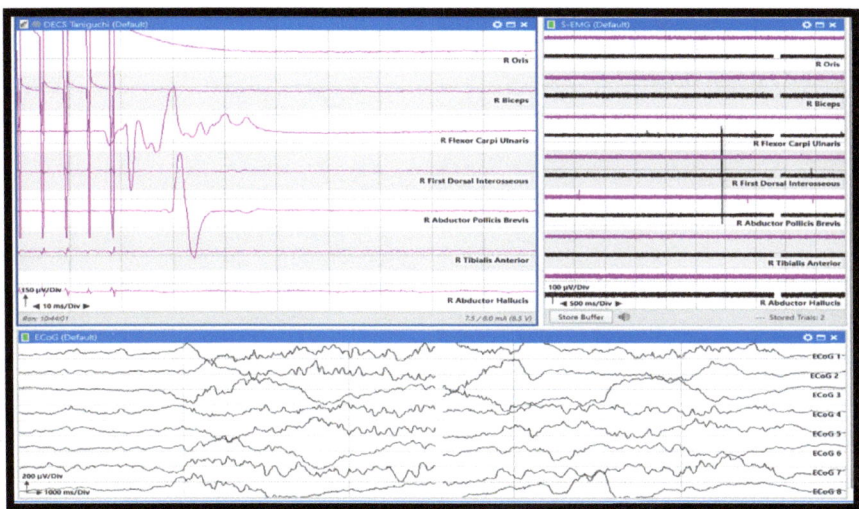

Figure 3: Taniguchi Method. High-Frequency Motor Mapping. *Top left:* motor mapping responses from right flexor carpi ulnaris and abductor pollicis brevis muscles. *Top right:* spontaneous electromyogram (EMG) responses contralateral muscles.

Bottom: Electrocorticography (ECoG) recordings from a 1x8 grid.

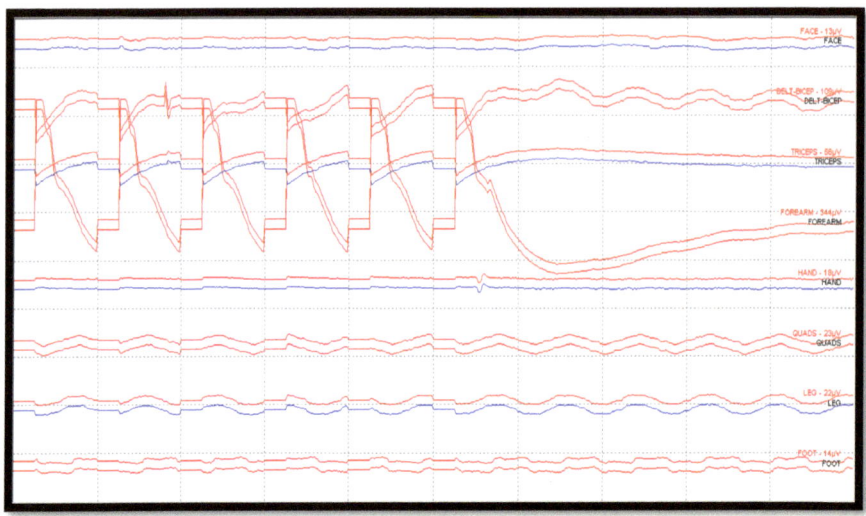

Figure 4: Penfield method: Slow frequency motor mapping. Motor mapping responses from deltoid, triceps, and forearm (flexor carpi ulnaris and brachioradialis) muscles.

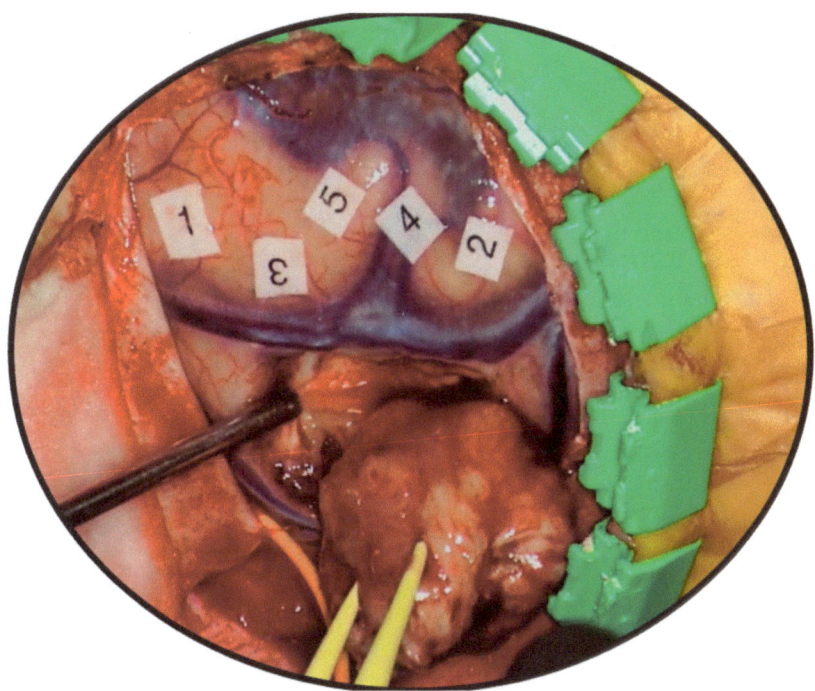

Figure 5: Motor Cortex. After localization and verification of the exact location of the motor areas, the tumor was resected. The patient underwent continuous awake testing of the right upper and lower extremity motor function. Papers marked with 1, 2, 3, 4, and 5 represent various cortical functional areas.

Language mapping (By DECS): After localization of the central sulcus and motor mapping, language mapping is performed by DECS and ECoG. DECS is performed by the Penfield method using hand-held bipolar ball tips probe with a monophasic or biphasic pulse duration of 0.5-1.0 milliseconds (ms) at a frequency of 50 Hz. The stimulation is applied for three to five seconds at each site. During stimulation, the subdural grid electrodes are positioned close to the stimulation sites to monitor ECoG for the presence of ADs or seizure activity. The stimulation is initiated at an intensity of 2.0 mA and increased as needed until a positive response (speech arrest/slurring) or After Discharges (ADs) were elicited or until clinical seizure activity was encountered (with a maximum limit of 15 mA for biphasic stimulation) (Fig 2). If ADs are present after DECS, ice saline (4°C) must be applied immediately to the exposed cortical surface to stop the ictal activity.

For each stimulated site, the patient is tested for various language tasks to evaluate brain function. The tests include reading sentences, auditory comprehension, visual comprehension, and spontaneous speech (Table 3). A positive mapping is a stimulation-induced language disruption in the absence of ADs. If there is a lack of stimulation-induced language disruption, it will be labeled as negative mapping. The frontal language sites are more predictable, and the temporal sites are variable. The language areas can be successfully identified in patients with gliomas. Language tasks such as number counting, object naming, and reading are performed during language mapping of the frontal and temporal lobes. The cortical areas are identified as a positing mapping if the patient cannot count, repeat words, read words, or name objects in two out of three stimulations. Speech arrest can be the result of language function disturbance and motor function disturbance. All cortical areas with positive mapping, vasculature, and subcortical white matter tracts must be preserved during resections.

The resection is then performed in these patients, repeating the same task, and a margin of 1 cm around the identified language areas is left. The resection of the cerebral tumors is performed if they show no language task deficits during electrical stimulation. The subcortical motor mapping can also be achieved by monopolar cathodal stimulation or bipolar stimulation.

There are some challenges when performing language mapping in awake patients. If the patient has a soft voice, it is recommended to use a microphone to amplify the sound volume. The sedation should be reduced if the patient is falling asleep during the mapping part. If the patient is getting tired, start the mapping from the most critical part. A soaked swab can help the patient if the patient complains about a dry mouth.

Counting: (Broca)
- Count from 1 to 20
- Count from 1 to 20 by 2s
- Count from 20 to 1

Days of the week: (Broca)
- Name the days of the week from Sunday
- Name the days of the week from Thursday

Name of the month: (Broca)
- Name the months from January
- Name the months from May

Alphabet: (Broca)
- Start from A
- Start from M

Noun: (Broca)
- Name 3 utensils you eat with
- Name 3 fruits
- Name 3 colors

Verb: (Broca)
- What do you do in a pool?
- What do you do with a book?
- What do you do with soap?

Object Naming: (ITLA)
- Flash card objects – nouns
- Flash card of actions – verbs

Sentence Completion (Wernicke - STG)
- A pilot flies an _____
- The color of grass is _____
- The news comes on at _____

Table 3: Language Mapping. Tasks for Language Mapping

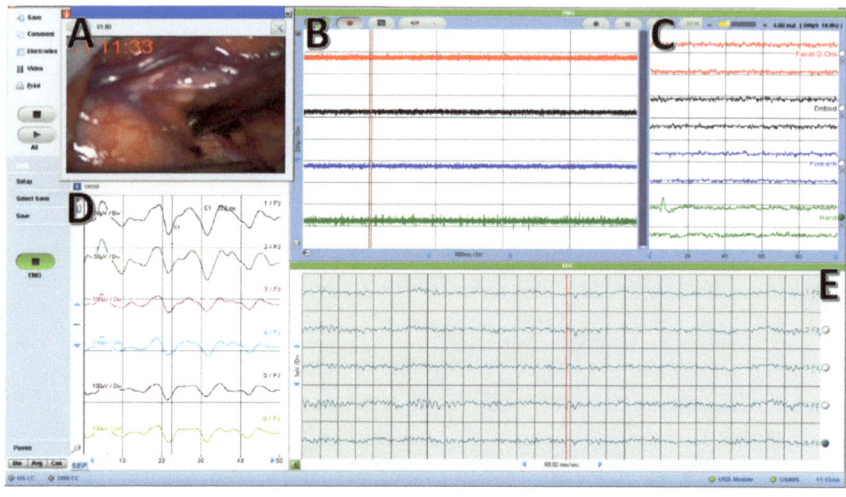

Figure 6: Intraoperative Neurophysiological Language Mapping (INLM). Intraoperative recordings during a language mapping awake craniotomy. (A) Video input from the microscope showing the cortex. (B) Spontaneous ELectromyogram (EMG). (C) DECS - Direct Electrical Cortical Stimulation. (D) Median nerve Phase Reversal (PR) window. (E) ELectrocorticography - ECoG.

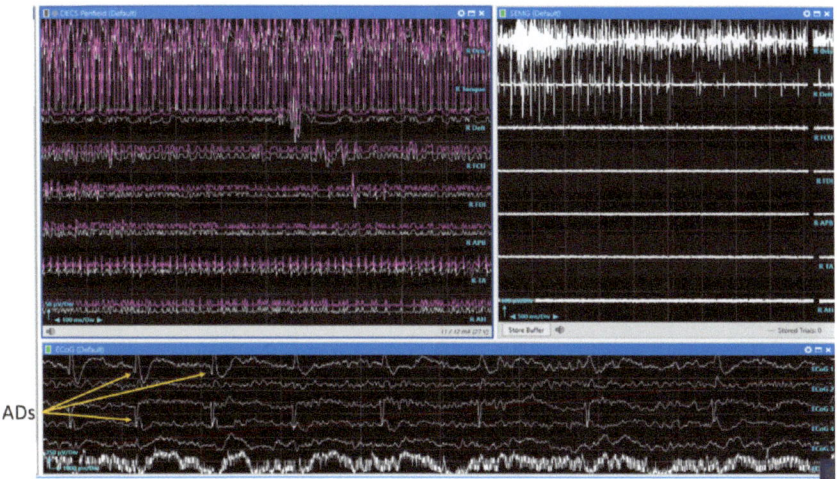

Figure 7: Intraoperative Neurophysiological Language Mapping (INLM). Language Mapping. Intraoperative recordings during a language mapping awake craniotomy. (Left upper) DECS - Direct Electrical Cortical Stimulation with responses from orbicularis oris and tongue muscles. (Right upper) Spontaneous ELectromyogram (EMG). (C) ELectrocorticography - ECoG with After Discharges (ADs) present after direct cortical motor stimulation (orange arrows).

Discussion:

The focus of neurology was once restricted to the conception of a holistic error within the brain tissue (encompassing the entire brain) or the behavior of a person being entirely separate from the brain's functioning. In combining his research on epilepsies and disconnection syndromes with his readings of Wernicke, Geschwind found a complex and multilayered explanation for aphasias that implicated lesions located in association pathways; when severe, these would cause behavioral disorders such as aphasias. The behavioral evaluation consists of a practice called awake craniotomy [7]. It effectively determines the functional ability to retain/possess linguistic functioning before, during, and after a procedure. This behavioral analysis prevents the cortex's unknowing lesioning of critical language areas through neural/behavioral monitoring.

Since the 1930s, surgeons and researchers could stimulate the brain directly. In recent years, intraoperative cortical stimulation has been adopted to identify and preserve language function and motor pathways during surgery. We have a limited understanding of the mechanism of stimulation effects on language. The principle is based upon local neurons' depolarization and passing pathways, local excitation or inhibition, and possible orthodromic or antidromic propagation to more distant areas. Such stimulation might be performed to determine the focus of epileptic seizures in a specific patient but can be used for linguistic cortex mapping.

Language mapping techniques were initially developed in the context of operations for treating epilepsy surgically. Large-scale craniotomies exposed the brain well beyond the region of surgical interest to localize multiple cortical regions containing stimulation-induced language areas to resection. These are termed "positive sites." Positive sites consist of neurons that respond to a small electric voltage with spreading cortical activation and linguistic disruption during analyses (observed during behavioral reading/reciting tasks). Researchers have been able to identify positive language sites in 95-100% of a given experimental sample [8]. Negative mapping is defined as directing resection by local cortical regions which contain no stimulation exerted by known language-related areas. Negative mapping becomes relevant in the absence of identified positive sites. By using negative sites, surgeons can reduce the cortical exposure necessary, increasing patient safety and efficiency. Determining the positive and negative sites of neural tissue cortically is discussed further.

Classical anatomical standards are insufficient to predict the location of language areas accurately. Variability of localization among individuals is one of the most consistent literature findings [7]). Therefore, the boundaries of language areas are not well defined. Language-associated activity has even been found in the primary motor cortex and the Sylvian fissure. There are interlobar differences in cortical excitability [3]. The temporal language area threshold is 1.5 higher than the threshold of the frontal language cortex. If there is a lesion near the language cortex, the threshold is increased 2.6 times. The edema in the language cortex's proximity increases its threshold by 1.8 times [9].

It is not possible to find the positive language sites before resection. Despite negative brain mapping, permanent postoperative neurologic deficits have been reported. This suggests the identification of negative sites may not be sufficient for limiting postoperative deficits. For example, a study of patients who underwent a glioma resection showed the patients with permanent postoperative neurologic deficits neglected to have had identified positive sites. (Loftus, 2014) This information would lend itself to a conclusion purporting the necessity of mapping for positive sites and negative sites.

In the recent literature, approximately 90 publications examine the utility of intraoperative stimulation mapping techniques in achieving a greater extent of resection for gliomas while minimizing morbidity. Within these studies, cohorts varied between 20 and 648 patients, with a median of 50 patients per study. Nearly all the reports provide level III evidence supporting microsurgical adjunct, except for two randomized studies that examined anesthetic and fluorescence-guided techniques to maximize the extent of resection [8]. Whereas pre-and intraoperative mapping and monitoring of motor and language function have already been established, the possibilities of neuropsychological or cognitive mapping and monitoring should be investigated more intensely. Neuropsychological testing before, during, and after glioma surgery should always be performed [10-12].

Currently, glioma resection operations using intraoperative neural monitoring have provided the most positive evidence for the technologies. Surgeons have reported the surgeries as having been more efficient, certainly more effective, and prolonged survival rates. Motor evoked potential recordings during surgery have been evidenced to prevent maladaptive cortical changes and increase tumor resection percentages.

Conclusion:

Intraoperative language mapping with cortical and subcortical stimulation is a reliable method for awake glioma resection surgery near functional pathways. In some patients, it may be beneficial to stimulate at a higher intensity at each cortical site regardless of the adjacent cortical areas' threshold. Resection with language mapping is associated with minimal postoperative neurologic deficits in language and speech functions. Determination of the improvement in preoperative language deficits and the duration of the postoperative deficits depends on the distance of the resection margin from the language sites. If the distance of the resection margin from the nearest language site is > 1 cm, significantly fewer permanent language deficits will occur. Cortical stimulation mapping for identifying essential language sites in patients with gliomas of the dominant hemisphere temporal lobe will maximize the extent of tumor resection and minimize permanent language deficits.

References:

1. Dineen J, Nahed BV, Simon MV: Mapping and monitoring of language and parietal functions. Intraoperative Neurophysiology: A comprehensive guide to monitoring and mapping. Mirela V. Simon (ed): Springer, 2019. Second:284-302.

2. Huncke K, Van de Wiele B, Fried I, Rubinstein EH: The asleep-awake-asleep anesthetic technique for intraoperative language mapping. Neurosurgery. 1998, 42:1312-6. 10.1097/00006123-199806000-00069

3. Pouratian N, Cannestra AF, Bookheimer SY, Martin NA, Toga AW: Variability of intraoperative electrocortical stimulation mapping parameters across and within individuals. J Neurosurg. 2004, 101:458-66. 10.3171/jns.2004.101.3.0458

4. Jahangiri FR: Surgical Neurophysiology: A Reference Guide to Intraoperative Neurophysiological Monitoring (IONM). Second Edition. CreateSpace, Charleston, SC, USA; 2012.

5. Jahangiri FR, Pautler K, Watters K, Anjum SS, Bennett GL: Mapping of the Somatosensory Cortex. Cureus. 2020, 12:10.7759/cureus

6. Jahangiri FR, Dobariya A, Kruse A, Kalyta O, Moorman JD: Mapping of the Motor Cortex. Cureus. 2020, 12:10.7759/cureus.10645

7. Kushner HI: Norman Geschwind and the Use of History in the (Re)Birth of Behavioral Neurology. Journal of the History of the Neurosciences. 2015, 24:173-192. 10.1080/0964704X.2014.950094

8. Loftus CM, Biller J, Baron EM: Intraoperative Neuromonitoring. McGraw-Hill Medical, New York; 2013.

9. Wang SG, Eskandar EN, Kilbride R, Chiappa KH, Curry WT, Williams Z, Simon MV: The variability of stimulus thresholds in electrophysiologic cortical language mapping. J Clin Neurophysiol. 2011, 28:210-6. 10.1097/WNP.0b013e3182121827

10. Ottenhausen M, Krieg SM, Meyer B, Ringel F: Functional preoperative and intraoperative mapping and monitoring: increasing safety and efficacy in glioma surgery. Neurosurgical Focus. 2015, 38:E3. doi:10.3171/2014.10.focus14611

11. Cervenka MC, Boatman-Reich DF, Ward J., Franaszczuk PJ, Crone NE: Language Mapping in Multilingual Patients: Electrocorticography and Cortical Stimulation During Naming. Frontiers in Human Neuroscience . 2011, 5:13. 10.3389/fnhum.2011.00013

12. Saito T, Muragaki Y, Maruyama T, Tamura M, Nitta M, Okada Y: Intraoperative Functional Mapping and Monitoring during Glioma Surgery. Neurologia Medico-Chirurgica. 2015, 55:1-13. doi:10.2176/nmc.ra.2014-0215

MAPPING OF THE BRAIN

MAPPING OF THE BRAIN

CONTRIBUTORS

Aaron Kruse
Graduate Student
Dept. of Neuroscience
School of Behavioral and Brain Sciences
The University of Texas at Dallas
Richardson, Texas

Aksharkumar Dobariya
Graduate Student
Dept. of Neuroscience
School of Behavioral and Brain Sciences
The University of Texas at Dallas
Richardson, Texas

Arshad Ali, MBBS, FCPS, MSc, FINR
Dept. of Neurosurgery
Neuroscience Institute
Hamad Medica Corporation
Doha, Qatar

Gurtegh S. Chima
Graduate Student
Dept. of Neuroscience
School of Behavioral and Brain Sciences
The University of Texas at Dallas
Richardson, Texas

Faisal R. Jahangiri, MD, CNIM, DABNM, FASNM, FASET
Vice President of Clinical Affairs
Axis Neuromonitoring LLC
Richardson, Texas

President
American Society of Neurophysiological Monitoring (ASNM)

Lecturer
Dept. of Neuroscience
School of Behavioral and Brain Sciences
The University of Texas at Dallas
Richardson, Texas

President/CEO
Global Innervation LLC
Dallas, Texas

Gabrielle L. Bennett
Graduate Student
Dept. of Neuroscience
School of Behavioral and Brain Sciences
The University of Texas at Dallas

Richardson, Texas

Jacob Jackson
Graduate Student
Dept. of Neuroscience
School of Behavioral and Brain Sciences
The University of Texas at Dallas
Richardson, Texas

John D. Moorman
Graduate Student
Dept. of Neuroscience
School of Behavioral and Brain Sciences
The University of Texas at Dallas
Richardson, Texas

Katharine Pautler
Graduate Student
Dept. of Neuroscience
School of Behavioral and Brain Sciences
The University of Texas at Dallas
Richardson, Texas

Keri Watters
Graduate Student
Dept. of Neuroscience
School of Behavioral and Brain Sciences
The University of Texas at Dallas
Richardson, Texas

Martha Pearson
Graduate Student
Dept. of Neuroscience
School of Behavioral and Brain Sciences
The University of Texas at Dallas
Richardson, Texas

Olga Kalyta
Graduate Student
Dept. of Neuroscience
School of Behavioral and Brain Sciences
The University of Texas at Dallas
Richardson, Texas

ABOUT THE AUTHOR

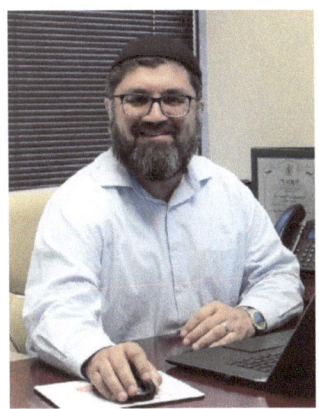

Dr. Faisal R. Jahangiri is the current President of the American Society of Neurophysiological Monitoring (ASNM) and working as a Vice President of Clinical Affairs at Axis Neuromonitoring LLC in Richardson, Texas. Dr. Jahangiri specializes in the field of Intra Operative Neurophysiological Monitoring (IONM). He has been teaching IONM courses at The University of Texas at Dallas (Texas) and Labouré College (Massachusetts). He is one of the few board-certified diplomates by the American Board of Neurophysiological Monitoring (ABNM).

Dr. Jahangiri graduated from Khyber Medical College, Peshawar, Pakistan, in 1991. After completing medical school and his general surgery and radiology training, he did his post-graduate studies in Biomedical Engineering at Case Western Reserve University in Cleveland, Ohio. His research included Functional Electrical Stimulation (FES), EEG, and 3-D imaging for reconstructive plastic surgery. Over the past two decades, he has worked as a senior clinical neurophysiologist and trainer with some premier IONM companies in the United States. He has also worked as a Consultant Clinical Neurophysiologist in the Division of Neurology, Dept. of Medicine at King Abdul-Aziz Medical City, Riyadh, Saudi Arabia, and as a Senior Consultant in the Department of Neurosurgery, Neuroscience Institute at Hamad Medical Corporation (HMC) in Doha, Qatar.

Dr. Jahangiri has monitored and supervised more than

9000 surgical procedures in more than 300 hospitals across 20 states in the USA, Middle East, and Pakistan. His expertise includes research, education, setting up new IONM programs, onsite supervision, and remote monitoring for neurosurgical, orthopedic, otolaryngology (ENT), vascular, general surgeries, as well as interventional procedures, intensive care units (ICU), and epilepsy monitoring units (EMU). He was awarded a fellowship by the ASNM in May 2013 (FASNM) and by the American Neurodiagnostic Society in Aug 2019 (FASET).

Dr. Jahangiri is also actively involved in the ASNM education, research, membership, and guideline committees. He was the chairman of the ASNM membership and awards committee from 2013-19, a board member since 2016, and currently President of ASNM. Dr. Jahangiri also offers an industry internship program in IONM for interested UTD students. He has more than 80 research publications, book chapters, and a regular guest speaker and course director at various national and international conferences. He has published two books, the second edition of an IONM reference book (*Surgical Neurophysiology*) and Mapping of the Brain.

MAPPING OF THE BRAIN

MAPPING OF THE BRAIN

www.ingramcontent.com/pod-product-compliance
Lightning Source LLC
Chambersburg PA
CBHW040320220526
45473CB00009B/2507